KW-222-062

Prai

"Dr Kaye is my GP and over the years, she has proved to be empathetic, interested and straight-talking. She's the mate who's always got your back; she knows her stuff and tells you exactly how it is. In this book she walks you through the maze of the menopause, and guides you through all the twists and unexpected turns your menopausal journey will take you on. Talking about periods is no longer done in hushed tones – my teenage daughter and I loudly discuss her period and her little brother knows all about them – we need to achieve that openness around the subject of menopause, and this book is a very good place to start."

**Sara Cox**

"An excellent read on everything you need to know about the menopause – informative, easy to digest and well balanced."
**Dr Sara Kayat, resident GP for *This Morning***

"I'll be recommending this book to my patients – an eminently sensible and evidence-based guide for everyone to understand the menopause."
**Dr Ellie Cannon, GP and *The Mail on Sunday* columnist**

"Contains positive and uplifting advice to help you understand the menopause, from the symptoms to expect to how to manage relationships."
*Hello!*

SOUTHWARK LIBRARIES

**SK 2879953   4**

"A taboo-busting medical guide to every aspect to the menopause, from coping with symptoms and treatment options to staying on top of work."
**Mail on Sunday**

"Every generation has a go-to practical classic: my grandmothers had Mrs Beeton, my mother's generation had Delia Smith, and now we have The M Word by Dr Philippa Kaye. This is the book I wish I'd read in my 20s (I'm 48 and postmenopausal)."
**Helen Kemp, Menopause Café Trustee**

"Based on the latest medical evidence and peppered with anecdotes, this one-stop guide is written by a GP with a special interest in women's and sexual health. It explains all, from understanding your symptoms to how the menopause and the years leading up to it can affect your work and sex life as well your relationships. There's lots of information on the pros and cons of HRT and other solutions that might help. In short, The M Word proves you can not just survive but thrive during menopause."
**Waitrose Weekend**

"Brilliant book."
**Red**

"An excellent, straight-talking guide to the menopause."
**Menopause Exchange**

"Frank, accessible and feminist answers to your medical questions."
**Grazia**

# THE

# M

# WORD

THE M WORD

This updated and expanded edition copyright © Dr Philippa Kaye, 2023
First published in 2020

All rights reserved.

No part of this book may be reproduced by any means, nor transmitted, nor translated into a machine language, without the written permission of the publishers.

Dr Philippa Kaye has asserted her right to be identified as the author of this work in accordance with sections 77 and 78 of the Copyright, Designs and Patents Act 1988.

Condition of Sale
This book is sold subject to the condition that it shall not, by way of trade or otherwise, be lent, resold, hired out or otherwise circulated in any form of binding or cover other than that in which it is published and without a similar condition including this condition being imposed on the subsequent purchaser.

An Hachette UK Company
www.hachette.co.uk

Vie Books, an imprint of Summersdale Publishers Ltd
Part of Octopus Publishing Group Limited
Carmelite House
50 Victoria Embankment
LONDON
EC4Y 0DZ
UK

www.summersdale.com

Printed and bound by CPI Group (UK) Ltd, Croydon, CR0 4YY

ISBN: 978-1-80007-831-4

Substantial discounts on bulk quantities of Summersdale books are available to corporations, professional associations and other organizations. For details contact general enquiries: telephone: +44 (0) 1243 771107 or email: enquiries@summersdale.com.

The author and the publisher cannot accept responsibility for any misuse or misunderstanding of any information contained herein, or any loss, damage or injury, be it health, financial or otherwise, suffered by any individual or group acting upon or relying on information contained herein. None of the views or suggestions in this book is intended to replace medical opinion from a doctor who is familiar with your particular circumstances. If you have concerns about your health, please seek professional advice.

Foreword by Vanessa Feltz

FULLY
REVISED &
UPDATED

# THE

# M

## WORD

EVERYTHING YOU NEED TO
KNOW ABOUT THE MENOPAUSE

# Dr Philippa Kaye

*For all the women in my life: my mother, my sisters,*
*my daughter and many more family and friends…*

# CONTENTS

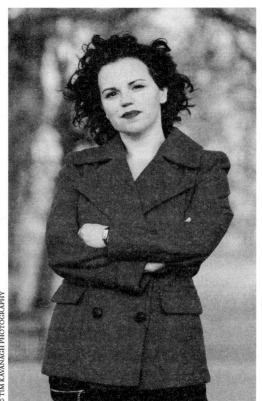

© TIM KAVANAGH PHOTOGRAPHY

# ABOUT THE AUTHOR

———◆———

**Dr Philippa Kaye MBBS (Hons), MA Hons (Cantab), MRCGP (2009), DCH, DRCOG, DFSRH** is a London-based GP with a particular interest in women's, children's and sexual health. She has been a GP for over a decade in both the NHS and private sectors. In addition to her general medical and GP qualifications, she holds the Diploma of the Royal College of Obstetrics and Gynaecology, the Diploma of the Faculty of Sexual and Reproductive Healthcare as well as the Diploma of Child Health (from the Royal College of Paediatrics and Child Health). She has written multiple books on women's and children's health and contributes to the national press, with weekly magazine columns and frequent newspaper quotes. She is also one of the UK's most well known and trusted media medics, regularly broadcasting on radio and television. Her general practice clinics are often filled with women seeking help for menopausal symptoms, or those not realizing that their symptoms could be related to the menopause, proving the need for a book dedicated to the menopause!

# Note to the reader:

This second edition of *The M Word* is bigger than the first; it covers even more symptoms and how to manage them. It includes tools to help you track your symptoms and is up to date with the latest information and newly available treatments, as well as being packed with practical advice. This really, absolutely is: "Everything you need to know about the menopause!"

# FOREWORD TO
# FIRST EDITION
# (FEBRUARY 2020)

———◆———

Menopause is the last taboo. Lord knows why, but it is shrouded in a conspiracy of silence. Grandmothers don't pass their Change of Life experiences on to their granddaughters. Mums keep mum. Sisters don't utter a syllable to their siblings. Best friends chat away about the most intimate details of their private lives but never their feelings about mood swings, disturbed sleep patterns or lost fertility. In 2020, most women cheerfully confide in one another about sex, money, disappointing husbands and challenging children. Occasionally we even opine about Brexit. What we do not do, under any circumstances, is mention the "M" word. We don't talk about our hot flushes. We don't discuss the dip in our desire or total extinction of our sex drives. We don't gossip about memory loss, night-time panic or feelings about our mortality.

We have no legacy of information to draw upon, so we all plunge into menopause in a state of unprepared shock. We vaguely know it will happen to us at some dreaded moment in the future. We just haven't the faintest idea of how to cope when it strikes.

That's why Dr Philippa Kaye's book is such a blessing. Philippa's warmth and wisdom fills the vacuum left by our non-communicative mums and grandmas. She steps in where no one else has dared to tread and tells us everything we badly need to know about menopause but were much too dazed and confused to ask. What's more, she's not just the understanding female relative we all wish we had – she also happens to be a doctor! We can trust her. She's impeccably informed but easy to understand and she has all bases covered. You really haven't lived until you've digested the chapter on sex which starts with what to do if you'd rather lag the loft than get down and dirty with your Other Half, and ends with a detailed description of the most gratifying sex toys!

My mother passed away at the age of 57. I'm 57 now. We'd never, not even once, broached the subject of the menopause. If you want to make sure your daughters and granddaughters approach the inevitable armed with the most up-to-date and easily absorbed information, secure in the knowledge that they won't be left to suffer miserably through the menopause, read this book and buy a copy for your friends, neighbours and descendants.

By the way, this isn't a female-only volume. Gentlemen, you won't escape scot-free. You'll have to endure the menopause by proxy. Peruse these pages and you'll be able to empathize, sympathize and you'll understand why she wants to sleep with all the windows open and a light smattering of snow on top of the duvet.

This is the book I wish I'd been given when the first symptoms of menopause struck. It will bring you confidence, clarity and consolation when you need it most.

With love and sisterly solidarity,

Vanessa Feltz

# INTRODUCTION

———◆———

The MP Rachel Maclean launched a menopause awareness campaign in June 2018, where she quoted an instagrammer @hotflush whose view was that menopause is "the club that no one wants to join". Ms Maclean MP further explained that "because no one wants to join it, no one on the outside has a clue what is going on inside". As with any taboo, the key is to start, and then to keep talking about it. This book will represent the "inside", to explain both to those in the club and those who are not what the menopause is and how to thrive while going through it. After all, half the population will go through the menopause and the other half is likely to be affected by it, due to the impact on the women in their lives, so men need to be informed too!

Most of what you hear and read about the menopause is, quite frankly, pretty dire and depressing. Not only are you beyond the point of childbearing, and therefore past the point of usefulness in what remains a patriarchal society where your main purpose as a female is apparently to bear children; but you are dripping with sweat, exhausted from insomnia and bouncing between being tearful and biting someone's head off. Add to this some wrinkly skin, a spare tyre round your tummy and a burgeoning moustache and it really isn't any wonder that many women dread the onset of the menopause. In the words of the rather fabulous Bette Midler, "it is true in this culture, they throw you out when you get older".

In May 2018, the Deputy Governor of the Bank of England described the economy as "menopausal", explaining his use of the word as a metaphor for something "past their peak and no longer so potent". While the Deputy Governor issued an apology for his statement, apologizing for its "ageist and sexist overtones", his use of the phrase is indicative of social attitudes towards the menopause, and not just for society as a whole but for women who do fear this stage in their lives. Many women see the menopause as the end and not a beginning; in all aspects of their lives, both physical and psychological, women seem to feel that they will be "all dried up". Yet this simply does not have to be the case.

## Let's talk about the menopause

If at some point you had the big talk – when someone told you about the birds and the bees, or your periods – why aren't we talking about the menopause? Hopefully this will begin to change as it was announced in 2019 that the menopause will be included in the personal, health, social and economic education curriculum in schools. With modern treatments and evidence-based knowledge we could view the menopause as the start of a new phase of life; women just need to know about it and the treatments for any symptoms that they may have. Put simply, you do not need to suffer, you do not need to "just about" manage, to just hang on in there, when we have treatments that can help.

An Ipsos MORI poll in 2016 on behalf of the British Menopause Society surveyed women between the ages of 45 and 65 who had been through the menopause in the previous ten years. This showed that women reported an average of seven menopause-related symptoms, with 42% saying that those symptoms were more severe than they had expected, as well as many women reporting symptoms that they had not expected such as sleeping problems or joint pains. Yet only half of the women surveyed saw a doctor or other healthcare professional for advice, support or treatment. A *Woman's Hour* poll in 2018 reported that 70% of women didn't have a strong understanding of the menopause, with only a third reporting a change in their mental health to their GP.

Half of the women surveyed said that their symptoms had impacted on their home lives, while 45% said that their menopausal symptoms affected and negatively impacted on their work lives. Yet just under half of women who needed to take a day off work due to their symptoms reported that they would not tell their employers the reason for their absence. Just over half reported an impact on their sex lives, with symptoms including loss of libido and painful sex, and one in ten had stopped having sex altogether. Social lives were also affected, with approximately a third of women reporting feeling less outgoing than before in social situations, or that they were no longer good company, and approximately one in four felt more isolated than before. And the effects didn't stop with the women themselves: approximately four out of ten men reported that they felt helpless as to how to support their partners through the menopause and three out of ten said that this could result in arguments at home.

These numbers haven't improved. The Fawcett Society produced a report in 2022 after surveying over 4,000 women which showed that over three quarters of women found at least one menopause symptom "very difficult" and over four out of ten women had at least three symptoms of this severity. The most common symptoms were insomnia, brain fog and anxiety or depression. Despite this, 45% of these women had not sought advice from their doctor, and many reported that they had not received the support they needed even when they did ask for help.

It is clear that the menopause is not simply about the periods stopping, but a myriad of symptoms that can affect all aspects of life.

In the UK, the average age when the menopause hits is 51 years old, but the average life expectancy for females is 81. This means that a third of the average woman's life is postmenopause. So we as women, and those around us, need to change our attitudes towards this stage to ensure that we can keep being who we are, being productive, being sexual, being happy. The menopause does not have to mean the end of relationships, libido, of sex, of work, of feeling like your "old self". You are still who you are – let's value that, let's celebrate that, let's honour that.

When the first edition of *The M Word* was published in February 2020, none of us could have predicted the events that followed; the coronavirus pandemic, multiple lockdowns, the cost-of-living crisis and far more. In the background of these seismic global changes, there have been developments regarding the perimenopause and menopause. Awareness is increasing and there have been various documentaries, radio and news coverage and countless press articles around the topic. Celebrities and public figures are telling their own menopause stories and the conversation is getting louder.

In October 2021, a second reading of a Menopause (Support and Services) Bill took place in the Houses of Parliament, followed by the establishment of the UK Menopause Task Force. In July 2022, the government published its Women's Health Strategy, after a call for evidence in the previous year. One of the key areas identified was the menopause, where an ambition was stated that everyone should have access to care and support as well as to education around the menopause. Despite HRT prescriptions being free in Scotland and Wales, a government pledge for one annual prescription fee for HRT will not come into effect until at least spring 2023 in England. There have also been significant HRT shortages, with some forms of HRT being rationed to three-monthly prescriptions in order to ease supply. This means that, currently, some women are paying more than previously. The HRT supply crisis, although it helped to give greater prominence to the issues of perimenopause and menopause, has caused untold anxiety for many women. There are countless reports of women swapping and sharing medication, buying it from unreputable sites online and travelling to other countries solely to get HRT (see page 285 for information about the shortages and for further advice).

The number of prescriptions for HRT has more than doubled in the last five years and although this is mainly due to manufacturing and supply issues some blame increased demand for the shortages. However, the fact that the number of prescriptions has gone up so much is a good thing; it means that more women are getting the help that they need.

The combination of successful campaigning, raised awareness and the HRT supply crisis has led to many more articles, television and radio programmes, podcasts and more covering the menopause. Yet the backlash was not far behind. Articles I have written often received comments from women that can essentially be summarized as "I sailed through, stop making a fuss". Campaigners have been accused of terrifying younger women about what is to come. Indeed, 20–25% of women may not have symptoms of the menopause, but this leaves approximately 75–80% that will, and for some women these symptoms are extremely severe, to the extent that one in ten have thoughts of suicide. There is a very big difference between raising awareness and scaremongering. This conversation is about educating and empowering women, not frightening them. In fact, talking about the perimenopause and menopause gives the opportunity for younger people to see that help is available if needed, as well as positive role models for an active fulfilling life after the menopause – not terrifying them, rather inspiring them! After all, data suggests that we actually get happier as we get older, and one study suggests that postmenopausal women have a more positive view of menopause and beyond than do younger ones – so surely young people need to hear more from these women, not less? The menopause is not solely a female issue. Everyone knows someone who has been or will go through this time so we all need to be informed!

As research continues and science develops, so too the guidance around the menopause and its treatments may change. The National Institute for Clinical Excellence (NICE) advised in May 2022 that their guidance around the menopause is being reviewed and updated. The areas being assessed include the use of cognitive behavioural therapy (CBT) for menopause symptoms, the management of genitourinary syndrome of the menopause (see page 174), and the effect of HRT on health. The updated guidance is due to be published in August 2023.

Menopause campaigns continue to gain pace, with calls for free prescriptions for HRT in all areas; for a national HRT formulary, which is a list of NHS allowable prescribable medicines to ensure that everyone has access to the same treatments no matter where they live; for further education; and for more specialist menopause clinics. There is still work to be done!

## A note about HRT

HRT is a form of medication which aims to replace and maintain the hormones that generally fall around the time of the menopause. It always includes oestrogen, it will include progesterone if you have a womb and it can also include testosterone if needed. HRT is discussed with regard to treating symptoms all through the book, but in Part Two the focus is mainly on lifestyle and other measures to control your symptoms. The idea that HRT is dangerous and should be avoided is long out of date. This book aims to change that, and to give women a real understanding of risks and benefits – or really benefits over small risks – in order to empower them to ask for help and treatment. For a full explanation of HRT, how it works, how it is delivered, the potential benefits and risks, please refer to Part Three of the book.

## Lifestyle or medicine?

When it comes to menopausal symptoms, the lifestyle versus medicine debate continues to rumble away. But actually these should not be presented in opposition to each other, rather as complementary – lifestyle and medicine should work together. There is a hashtag on social media – #foodismedicine – which essentially oversimplifies the situation; we have always obtained medications from plants and herbs, and lifestyle factors absolutely have a role to play in both disease and in health. But food is not medicine, it does not replace medication, and while, for example, being a healthy weight by eating a healthy diet and exercising can help lower your blood pressure, you may also need medication to keep your blood pressure under control. In an ideal world, in this particular example the blood pressure medication would not be used instead of lifestyle measures, but in conjunction with them, if needed.

Wherever I have covered a symptom and the options for managing or treating it, I have included the lifestyle options, as well as a cross reference to any relevant medications, including HRT, which themselves are covered in detail in Part Three. Of course, I appreciate that many people would prefer to avoid medication if possible, and the lifestyle measures discussed will help you control and manage those symptoms, but if they do not, or if they are not enough, then please speak to your doctor to see what other treatment options are available for you. And on the other hand, having medication, be it in the form of HRT or something else, does not mean that you can ignore all the lifestyle modifications which are recommended, as many of these are preventative.

Let's get informed and become empowered to make our own choices about our symptoms, our treatments, our minds and our bodies. And then, let's keep talking – to our friends, to our families, to the men in our lives, to our children. Let's spread the word so that no woman feels alone or ashamed of this natural stage in her life.

# Part One

# ALL ABOUT THE MENOPAUSE

# CHAPTER 1:

# BACK TO SCHOOL

———◆———

Brace yourselves, here comes the science bit…

If the mention of the word "science" makes you break out in a sweat, reminding you of time spent on a stool in a high-school lab, don't worry: I am going to make this as simple as possible, so please don't just skip over this section! If you have some understanding of what is going on with your hormones around the time of the menopause, then you will be able to understand better the potential treatments and choose which ones you think may suit you. Knowledge is power! So scrape your hair back, pull on an imaginary white coat (or your school uniform) and let's enter the world of your hormones.

## It's all about hormones

The word "menopause" literally means "the last period". See, that was easy! However, we can't say that you have gone through the menopause until you haven't had a period for a year. The word for your first period is menarche, but the whole process of puberty – from growing breasts, hair and upwards to starting your periods – takes years, and so too does the period of change around the time of the menopause, called the perimenopause, climacteric or menopause transition.

Puberty is associated with lots of hormonal changes. The brain starts secreting a hormone called gonadotrophin-releasing hormone (GnRH), which then triggers another part of the brain to produce two further hormones, luteinizing hormone (LH) and follicle-stimulating hormone (FSH). The hormones work together to trigger the ovaries to produce oestrogen, progesterone and a small amount of testosterone, and these five hormones working together cause the changes of puberty.

Once your periods (your menstrual cycle) have started, multiple hormones from the brain and ovaries work together to keep your periods coming every month. Your ovaries are found in your pelvis, on either side of the womb, and are generally about the size of an egg – a chicken's egg, that is, not a goose egg or even a human one! So here we go, high-school biology coming up…

Day 1 of your menstrual cycle is day one of your period and we are going to start there. Even as you are menstruating, the part of your brain called the hypothalamus is already starting the next cycle by releasing GnRH. This in turn triggers another part of the brain, called the pituitary gland, to release follicle-stimulating hormone (FSH). Even though it is produced in the brain, FSH acts on the ovary and stimulates the development of one or more of the immature, undeveloped follicles (fluid-filled sacs which each contain an egg) in the ovary.

Still with me? Jolly good. So, the developing follicle gets bigger and the egg in it also grows and develops. Now, the cells around this follicle produce oestrogen, which has many effects in the body, but for the purposes of the menstrual cycle it acts on the lining of the womb, building it up gradually, so that if conception occurs, and a sperm has fertilized an egg, there is a nice thick lining for the egg to implant into.

So far, so good. The first half of your menstrual cycle is generally when you feel your best as a result of the rising oestrogen. The FSH and oestrogen levels gradually keep rising, and if you have a regular 28-day cycle, at about day 12–13 the pituitary gland in your brain responds to this rise by releasing a second hormone – luteinizing hormone (LH). This surge triggers ovulation and the mature egg pops out of the follicle. The length of this first, follicle phase decides the length of your menstrual cycle. Once ovulation occurs, your period will start in about 14 days. So if your cycle is 28 days you will ovulate at about day 14, if it is 33 days you will ovulate at about day 19.

We're not done quite yet. Now we have an egg but the shell of the follicle from which it emerged still has work to do. It is now called the corpus luteum and produces the hormone progesterone, which again has multiple effects in the body, but in the womb acts to mature that womb lining to ensure the best conditions for egg implantation.

Almost there, no falling asleep at the back! You will still be producing some oestrogen at this point and the oestrogen and progesterone work together to maintain that all-important lining for about a further week. But unless you conceive (and this is a book about menopause and perimenopause so I am going to assume this is not what we are after) the levels of both oestrogen and progesterone fall. This means that the lining of the womb becomes unstable and is shed, and voila – you have your period.

And then the whole lot starts again over and over, month on month, until you are pregnant, or get to the point of reading this book, which is when changes are beginning to happen again.

---

One more hormone to mention: testosterone. It is produced by the ovaries in much smaller amounts than is produced by the testes in men, but it is there and is important, especially for your libido, or sex drive.

---

# Eggs count

Men have the capacity to continue making sperm their entire lives; they can make women pregnant from puberty right until the end of life. But women have a finite number of eggs, already predetermined before the moment they are conceived and already reduced by the time they are born, though these initial eggs that you have when you are born and as a child are very premature. Although you have many, many more eggs than you will ever need – about 1–2 million or so – about 10,000 eggs die every month until you hit puberty and by the time you get there you have about 300,000–400,000 eggs left (though the thought of 400,000 children is enough to give most of us a bit of a turn!). From the moment when you start your periods onwards you lose about 1,000 eggs a month: not all of these develop and are released, the majority get reabsorbed. Only one (sometimes two to make twins) is released each month. Only about 500 follicles mature to release an egg, so if you have a period once a month that would give you about 40 years or so of regularly having periods.

Essentially, over time, the reserves of eggs in the ovaries are depleted, and this combined with the fact that the body selects the healthiest eggs earlier in life to ovulate, means that as you get older it is harder to become pregnant. A woman's fertility starts to decline quite rapidly after the age of 35. By societal standards this is still relatively young, but reproductively it isn't!

As the number of follicles in the ovaries that can produce and release eggs continues to fall around the time of the menopause, the oestrogen and progesterone levels also begin to fall. Now, the body responds to this by whacking up how much luteinizing hormone (LH) and follicle-stimulating hormone (FSH) it produces, trying harder and harder to make the ovaries produce eggs. Due to the lower levels of oestrogen and progesterone the lining of the womb doesn't build up so the periods may become irregular, further apart or even closer together until they eventually stop appearing at all.

Although 1–2 million eggs going down to virtually none may sound catastrophic, it is a natural and expected process in the body. However, for some women the menopause is brought on early, for example if they have had their ovaries removed surgically to treat cancer, or if the ovaries stop working due to chemotherapy, radiotherapy or other medications. The symptoms are the same whether or not the process was brought on by an operation or medication, or if it occurred naturally, though in a surgical or medical menopause they may be more severe (see Chapter 3 for more detailed information about premature menopause).

After the menopause your ovaries will still produce some oestrogen, though far less than before, and some testosterone. Postmenopausal levels of progesterone are undetectable. Fat cells in the body are also capable of producing oestrogen, though in a less potent way (the chemical term is oestrone which is produced from fat cells, compared to oestradiol which is more potent and produced by the ovaries), and the adrenal glands can also produce small amounts of testosterone. So you will still naturally be producing some hormones, though at a far lower level than previously.

And relax – all done. You all get an A★, or a level 9, or whatever they are using to grade exams at the moment. (Except you in the third row who gagged at the word ovary.) Later on, when you are reading about a diet rich in phytoestrogens, and about herbs, or about hormonal medications, pop back here if you need to remind yourself of the whys and hows as this may help you decide which treatments to try.

## The perimenopause

Think back to puberty. That whole process took quite a few years and so do the changes relating to the menopause. Teenagers are known for being "hormonal", and puberty is associated with huge psychological, mental and emotional changes. These changes are not just around the change in their bodies but also about their change in self, as they create and develop their own personalities and behaviours with increasing independence from their parents. The menopause and perimenopause also involve an enormous amount of hormonal and physical changes and yet we seem to be kinder and more understanding towards our teenagers (even our own children) than we, or society, are to ourselves when going through the menopause. The sex hormones oestrogen, progesterone and testosterone don't just act in the genitals, ovaries and womb, they act all over the body, from the breasts to the skin. If the sex hormones act everywhere, then it is understandable that the change in levels of these hormones can have wide-ranging signs and symptoms.

As mentioned above, from as early as your late 30s and early 40s, the ovaries start not to work as effectively as before. Interestingly, many women notice that their menstrual cycle gets slightly shorter by a few days, but this doesn't mean that the menopause is imminent. This period (sorry!) can last a decade or so and in it you may get symptoms which are attributable to the menopause, from changes to your periods to flushes and sweats and mood changes. And the decline in ovarian function isn't linear; they don't gradually stop working a little less each month. Instead they can work well one month and then not the next. This also means that your hormone levels, and therefore your symptoms, can fluctuate wildly too. But fear not! Even if you are having periods – regular, irregular or totally haywire – there are still treatments that can help control your symptoms.

## Menopause, weight and muscles

Loss of muscle mass occurs with ageing, starting as early as the 30s and 40s, and accelerates during the perimenopause and menopause. The role of your muscles is not exclusively related to movement and body strength and whether or not you can carry all your supermarket shop from your car to the fridge in one trip! Muscles have many roles; they are involved in your metabolism (how you convert food into energy) and produce anti-inflammatory chemicals in the body, as well as being involved in keeping your bones strong and healthy. Losing muscle mass is also associated with increased insulin resistance, meaning that the body doesn't respond well to insulin and needs to produce more to compensate.

Weight gain is common around the perimenopause and beyond and is thought to be related in part to the loss in muscle mass, which in turn leads to fewer calories burned and increased insulin resistance.

During the menopause, women are more likely to gain visceral fat, which is "hidden" fat around the internal organs such as the liver, as opposed to subcutaneous fat, which is elsewhere. Visceral fat leads to increased inflammation in the body and is metabolically active, in that it may influence hormone levels and is linked with higher cholesterol levels and insulin resistance (which may contribute to conditions such as diabetes and cardiovascular disease). This gain in visceral fat may be related to the loss of muscle mass or to the hormonal changes of the perimenopause and menopause. The best way to maintain muscle mass is through exercise, in particular, regular resistance-based exercise, both before the menopause and beyond. For more information about exercise and physical activity, and healthy eating see page 111.

## Menopause and the cardiovascular system

Before the menopause, cardiovascular disease (which includes heart attack and stroke) is more common in men. After the menopause, the gap between men and women with regard to cardiovascular disease shrinks. This may be due to lower levels of oestrogen or the increase in visceral fat that occurs during perimenopause and beyond and is associated with higher cholesterol and insulin resistance. To look after your heart and cardiovascular system, try to stop smoking, maintain a healthy weight, and move your body – for more information please see pages 111-119.

## Menopause and the brain

Oestrogen performs lots of functions within the brain such as increasing blood flow and improving brain connectivity (connections between different parts of the brain). It is involved in the production of serotonin, which has roles in mood and executive function and how well your brain can prioritize and work on tasks. This involves a combination of concentration, memory, thinking and self-control – after all it doesn't matter if you can concentrate on a task well if you don't have the self-control to start doing it! The brain is primed to respond to hormonal changes, for example after pregnancy. Before we all panic though, remember that your brain worked before puberty when there was less oestrogen, and that many women do not take HRT and can function as normal, or maybe even better than before when they were too exhausted perhaps from childcare or other demands, or distracted by period pains! It may also be that symptoms such as brain fog are temporary, and indeed many people report that their symptoms improve after some time, perhaps as the brain continues to rewire itself. As with protecting your heart and cardiovascular system, you can optimize your brain function by stopping smoking, eating a healthy balanced diet and keeping physically active.

# Why do we go through the menopause?

I can explain the science of what is happening at the time of the menopause, the change in your hormones and ovaries, and so on, but the purpose of the menopause is much harder to decipher. To put it in terms of an existential crisis, what is the point of it all? From an evolutionary point of view it is even harder to explain: if the point of life is to reproduce and pass on your genes, why continue to survive when you can no longer do so? And remember that this point where you may not be able to reproduce isn't even just after the menopause; in the years leading up to it your fertility declines rapidly. You can still be having periods, irregularly or regularly, but not be able to get pregnant in the years before the menopause (though for some it is still possible).

Interestingly, most mammals don't go through the menopause like we do. In general they are able to keep reproducing in older age, albeit at a reduced rate. In mammals that don't go through the menopause the chances of reproductive success decrease with age. Many fish, birds and invertebrates seem to go through a menopause – by that I am not saying their periods stop, as they don't have periods in the first place. They enter a post-reproductive stage in their lives, but they seem to die shortly afterwards. In fact, our closest genetic relatives – primates such as chimps – stop having babies in their late 30s and tend to die within a few years. Which is rather depressing. Yet human females live approximately one third of their lives after the menopause. And this isn't just in affluent countries.

So who is with us, going through the menopause and then living a substantial part of their lives afterwards? Other mammals who go through the menopause include two types of whales: the short-finned pilot whale and the killer whale. The latter generally goes through the menopause at about 40 years old, but they can live into their 90s.

So here we are, us and the killer whales, going through the menopause. A commonly held theory as to why this occurs is the "grandmother hypothesis", which holds that older women stop reproducing so they can help with rearing their children and grandchildren, thus ensuring the survival of their children and grandchildren and thereby their own genes. Even the whales appear to do grandparent childcare! But grandmothering and the menopause don't always occur together; for example, the family structure is hugely important in elephant communities, with the matriarchs playing a significant role, and yet they don't go through the menopause. And from a maths perspective, it doesn't add up – your own children are 50% genetically yours, but your grandchildren have only 25% of your genes, so wouldn't you want those with more of your genes to survive? I am of course taking emotion out of the equation!

Another reason may be competition for resources; after all, without food no one survives. If females of all ages are competing for food as they are reproducing and focusing solely on their own children, there would be less for all. From a human point of view, if both you and your daughter are having a baby at the same time and are competing for food, the chances of survival and therefore the survival of your genes decreases. And if you add to that the higher risks of miscarriage, foetal abnormality and complications during pregnancy and labour the older you (and therefore your eggs) become, perhaps, from an evolutionary standpoint, you are better off caring for the children you already have than trying to make more. Consider how families used to work (and in some areas still do): the sons would stay in the family group but the daughters would leave and join the husband's family, to whom they generally would have no genetic connection. Therefore a daughter would gain nothing (in purely genetic terms) by helping her own mother-in-law reproduce. But once she has children and grandchildren, she has now become genetically connected to her husband's side, perhaps increasing her desire to help them survive.

Perhaps it is the very fact that we go through a menopause that further divides us from primates and other mammals. Freed from the burdens of reproduction and child-rearing, we have time to do other things – be that gathering food or ruling the world! Rather than considering the menopause as a sign that we are "past it", perhaps it provides new opportunities for us to contribute to our family, community or wider society. It may in fact be nature's way of showing us that women *do* have value beyond youth and reproduction.

Or is it simply an effect of us living longer and that some bits wear out faster than others? Hundreds of years ago we simply wouldn't have lived particularly long after the menopause. Or is it a fluke and there is no particular evolutionary logic, grand meaning or reasoning behind it at all?

I can't answer what the point of it all is – no one can – in life, as well as in the menopause. But that doesn't mean that your life doesn't have a value, purpose or point after the menopause – you can now make your own!

## SUMMARY POINTS

- Menarche – the first period.
- Menopause – the last period.
- Climacteric – the time leading up to the last period, when hormone levels can go up and down, and the fluctuating levels can cause menopausal symptoms though you can still be having regular (or irregular) periods.
- Perimenopause – the time from the start of any menopausal symptoms (in the climacteric), all the way to the postmenopausal. Often though the terms climacteric and perimenopause are used interchangeably. We will use the term perimenopause throughout this book.
- Postmenopause – literally means "after the menopause". The menopause is a diagnosis of retrospect, in that we only say you are postmenopausal when you have not had a period for over one year. Alternatively, if you have had your ovaries removed there is no need to wait for 12 months as you will immediately be postmenopausal.
- The symptoms of the perimenopause and menopause are related to the change in hormone levels as the ovaries gradually stop producing eggs each month.

# CHAPTER 2:

# AM I THERE YET?

———◆———

*"As soon as I hit my early 40s, every time something happened my sister or friends would assume it was the menopause: boiling hot heatwave and I'm hot and sweaty, 'are you there yet?', grumpy after a hard day at work and kids driving me mad, 'are you there yet?', looking knackered at a dinner after a poor night's sleep, 'are you there yet?'. On and on 'are you there yet?', 'are you through yet?', 'are you there yet?'. It was like a weird version of that thing your kids do in the car when you have a two-hour journey and they start when you are just turning out of your own road 'are we there yet? Are we there yet? Are we there yet?' No!! Not yet, and for f\*ck's sake, stop asking!"*

Cassie, 49, not there yet

One of the questions I am most commonly asked about the perimenopause is "does (insert your symptom of choice) mean I am menopausal?". From a medical point of view, unless you have not had a period for over 12 months the answer is no, you are not. But that is not what these women are asking, they are asking if they are "going through the change", or in medical terms, in the perimenopause. And the answer to that is, if you are having symptoms relating to the menopause, most probably yes.

# When is it going to happen?

Unfortunately my crystal ball is broken and I can't tell you exactly when it will be as the timing is slightly different for everyone, but the average age for a woman in the UK to go through the menopause is 51. Remember, you can't say that you have been through the menopause until you haven't had a period for a year and you may have had symptoms for a good few years prior to that, but the average age is 51. This means that most women in the UK have their last period somewhere between about 49 and 53, though you may have had irregular periods for a while. As long as you are over 40 when your last period occurs this means you haven't had a premature menopause. Equally, there are no concerns if you go through it later – my oldest patient who is still having periods is currently 57!

When you will have your menopause is decided by a number of factors, mainly by the number of follicles (and therefore eggs) that you have. So at some point in the future we may well be able to predict this simply by counting follicles, though currently we cannot do so. The number of follicles you are born with and the timing of your menopause may have a genetic factor as it tends to be that women with family members who have had a late or early menopause often follow a similar pattern, though there is no guarantee of this. And potentially, starting your periods early – under the age of 12 – may increase the likelihood of an earlier menopause, though this cannot be just because more eggs are being used up earlier, as we have many thousands more than we need!

Certain medical conditions are also linked with an earlier menopause, though not necessarily a premature one; for example, it can be linked with autoimmune conditions such as type 1 diabetes, thyroid disease and rheumatoid arthritis.

Having a hysterectomy (surgery to remove the womb) also increases your risk of an early menopause, even if the ovaries are left alone. Women who have had a hysterectomy where the ovaries are left in place tend to go through the menopause two years earlier than those who have not.

Finally, medication and surgery to remove the ovaries can induce the menopause. There is more information about these triggers in Chapter 3, though if they occur over the age of 40, it is not considered a premature menopause.

Although the last period of the menopause itself is a moment in time, the perimenopause can begin as much as a decade earlier and symptoms can be present for years.

## Can I delay it?

Most of the factors that determine the timing of the onset of your menopause are set and unchangeable. After all, you can't go back in time and put more follicles into your ovaries. However, that doesn't mean that there is nothing that you can do:

◆ Stop smoking. Yes, you knew that I was going to say that – I am a doctor, after all! Of the myriad adverse effects that smoking has, one of them is that it can bring the menopause on earlier. On average, women who smoke go through the menopause approximately two years earlier than those who don't. Why? Smoking doesn't just affect your lungs, it affects your heart, brain and increases the risk of multiple cancers all over the body. Smoking helps fur up the arteries of the body, by being involved in a complex process called atherosclerosis, and narrowed, furred up arteries mean a reduced blood and therefore oxygen supply to your organs – and that includes the ovaries, leading to an earlier menopause. It can also make the symptoms of the menopause worse, though more on that later. Even regular exposure to second-hand smoke can lead to an increased risk of a slightly earlier menopause, so get nagging whoever it is to stop!

♦ Up your intake of oily fish, legumes, vitamin B6 and zinc. A study published in April 2018 in the *Journal of Epidemiology and Community Health* showed that women who ate oily fish (90 g per day), legumes (also 90 g per day) and have a higher intake of vitamin B6 and zinc have a later menopause. This study followed over 14,000 women, nearly 1,000 of whom went through the menopause during the four-year period of the study. Not only did it show that eating oily fish and legumes delayed the menopause, but for each increase in the amount of oily fish they ate the later it was, when compared with women who ate more rice and pasta. Oily fish such as salmon, trout, mackerel and sardines are rich in omega-3 fatty acids which have multiple health benefits. In this study it was shown that women who ate a vegetarian diet, despite having fresh legumes, had an earlier menopause than those who regularly ate oily fish. This may be that oily fish and legumes contain antioxidants which help prevent damage to the ovaries, though this is not conclusive. Eating at least two portions of oily fish a week with plenty of legumes is a healthy option in general and may affect the timing of your menopause. Worth a try!

♦ Ensure you're getting enough calcium and vitamin C. An earlier study in 2017 published in *The American Journal of Clinical*

*Nutrition* indicated that a diet low in calcium and vitamin D could lead to an earlier menopause. This doesn't mean that a diet high in calcium and vitamin D would delay the menopause and interestingly taking a calcium or vitamin D supplement doesn't seem to make a difference, so perhaps it is something else found in dairy.

◆ A new surgical procedure was reported in August 2019, whereby women have a piece of one of their ovaries removed in their 20s or 30s, which is then frozen until the women reach the menopause. At that point, the ovarian tissue is transplanted back and essentially starts working again, therefore delaying the menopause for a number of years. This is not a routinely available surgery, there is not evidence as yet for its efficacy and it doesn't delay the menopause indefinitely.

# Can I take a test to determine whether I am menopausal?

If only it were so simple – a blood test to give us a yes or no answer. But like most things related to the menopause, it is not quite as easy as that!

Remember from our science lesson in Chapter 1 that the decline in ovarian function is not linear; they don't gradually stop working a little less each month. Instead, one month they can be perfect, working efficiently and effectively, and the next not. This means that your hormone levels (and therefore your symptoms) can also fluctuate wildly. We can test the hormone levels, but the question is more whether or not we should. And if we should, when should we?

The hormones most generally tested are follicle-stimulating hormone (FSH) and luteinizing hormone (LH). Back to biology, the FSH levels rise to stimulate the ovaries to then produce oestrogen. As the oestrogen levels fall in the menopause the pituitary gland works harder than ever, pumping out more and more FSH to try to stimulate the ovaries back to work. And even within a particular month the FSH levels change. The best time to test would be day 2–5 of your menstrual cycle (remember that day 1 is the first day of your period), as at this point FSH levels tend to be at their lowest, so we possibly could get a baseline level. But even within those few days the levels can still fluctuate. And some of you will not be having regular enough periods to be able to book a blood test on the "correct" days.

This means that while you're in the perimenopause, the hormone test one month could say you are through the menopause and the next month say you are not, or even vary to that extent within the same month.

All in all, then, a single test is not likely to be very useful, unless your FSH levels are through the roof – say above 100 IU/L – but otherwise they don't tell us very much.

## So how do I know if I am in the perimenopause?

◆ If you are over the age of 45 – if you are having menopausal symptoms such as flushes, sweats, changes to your periods, then we don't need to do a test, for all the reasons set out above, you are in the perimenopause. (And again, don't worry we can help you, periods or not.) This means the perimenopause is a clinical diagnosis at this age, as it does not involve tests.

◆ If you are over the age of 45 and haven't had a period for a year you are through the menopause and are considered postmenopausal.

◆ If you are over 45 and you don't have a uterus – for example, if it was removed surgically – you don't have periods at all to guide us, so instead we rely on your symptoms.

◆ If you are under the age of 45 – here we need to check the hormone levels. "But you just said they don't work!" Yes I know, I know, but I also said things aren't simple! We can't rely on a single FSH test as the levels can fluctuate so wildly, instead we use two FSH blood tests taken six weeks apart. If the levels are over 30 IU/L on both occasions then you are considered to be menopausal.

And I still have a but: if you are on certain forms of hormonal contraception, such as the combined pill (which contains both oestrogen and progesterone), or high-dosage progesterone, the test won't give an accurate result and therefore isn't helpful. We will cover more about this when we look at contraception around the menopause in Chapter 8.

Other blood tests are neither helpful nor required at this point, including those that check the level of oestrogen, progesterone and others such as inhibin A, inhibin B and anti-mullerian hormone (AMH). AMH is a hormone which can give an indication of ovarian reserve – the capacity of the ovaries to produce an egg which could be fertilized. It can be used as part of fertility testing but it doesn't tell us if you are postmenopausal or when you are perimenopausal.

*"I went to my doctor for a test, I wanted to know, have I gone through the menopause or not? The doctor wouldn't give me one, said they didn't work. So I cried, the flushes were making me crazy, I couldn't sleep and I felt I was losing my mind. I didn't realize that I didn't need a test to have treatment, thankfully the doctor did!"*

Emily, 49

## SUMMARY POINTS

- The average age of a woman in the UK having her last period is 51 years old.
- Symptoms can occur before, during and after this point, whether or not you are having periods.
- Smokers tend to go through the menopause on average two years earlier than non-smokers.
- If you are over the age of 45, and have symptoms, blood tests are not needed to confirm if you are perimenopausal or menopausal.

# CHAPTER 3:

# AREN'T I TOO YOUNG FOR THIS?

———◆———

*"I was 38 and had two children, a full-time job, a dog, two cats, and an attempt at a social life. I was and am the busy one, which is exactly how I like it, with lots to do and people to see. So I was tired, and busy, and distracted and didn't really pay much attention to my periods. They were there, or not. And then I realized it had been a while, cue rush to do a pregnancy test, which was negative. But they didn't come back, I wasn't sleeping well and just didn't feel good. A blood test showed I was in the menopause, which was a huge shock. Though my mum then told me she was about 40 too. The doctor gave me HRT which has helped with the physical symptoms but I still felt a loss for a long time."*

Hannah, 44

If the menopause occurs before the age of 40 it is considered to be "premature menopause", which doctors call "premature ovarian insufficiency". It isn't uncommon. The menopause is thought to occur in about 5% of those under 45, occurring in one in 100 women under the age of 40. It can occur as early as the teens or 20s, though this is less common, with only one woman in 1,000 being diagnosed under the age of 30 and one in 10,000 under 20.

# What makes the menopause start earlier than expected?

*"My first thought was, why me?"*

Diane, 36

There are various known causes of a premature or early menopause, but in some cases no cause can be identified. However, it seems to run in families so there may be a genetic link, perhaps meaning that you had fewer eggs initially or they are reabsorbed quicker than expected.

## Primary causes

The periods didn't start, either because there were no ovaries, or the ovaries didn't develop properly or don't work. There are generally genetic reasons for this such as Turner's syndrome, which affects approximately one in 2,000 girls whereby instead of having two X chromosomes there is only one X chromosome, though autoimmune conditions can also be a cause.

## Secondary causes

The periods started but either became irregular and stopped, or are still present but there are other menopausal symptoms.

◆   Autoimmune conditions – an autoimmune condition is one where the body's immune system begins to attack itself, for example in type 1 diabetes and some thyroid diseases. Here, the antibodies seem to attack the ovaries.

- Infection – mumps after puberty can affect the ovaries, as can tuberculosis and malaria.
- Medical causes – such as chemotherapy and radiotherapy. Other medications can stop ovulation or the ovaries working while you are on them, but the ovaries tend to start functioning again when the medication is stopped.
- Surgical causes – removal of the ovaries will lead to a premature menopause. Even if the ovaries are left in place during a hysterectomy when the womb is removed, the menopause can begin earlier than average.

# Diagnosis of premature menopause

Women often don't get diagnosed with premature menopause until they are trying to conceive as they may get irregular periods in their early perimenopause or could be using forms of contraception such as the combined oral contraceptive pill that could mask the irregular or absent periods that could indicate early menopause because they mean that you bleed monthly (but this is a withdrawal bleed rather than a true period), or not bleed at all. The pill stops ovulation and the bleed is from the withdrawal of hormones in the pill-free interval, so unfortunately it doesn't give us an indicator of ovarian function, its whole purpose is to stop them working and producing eggs.

For women over the age of 45, blood tests to diagnose the menopause are not useful but they are used in the diagnosis of premature menopause. At a younger age, your doctor may request blood tests for other conditions that can affect your periods, such as thyroid or prolactin problems, as correcting these can allow the ovaries to start working again. The levels of follicle-stimulating hormone (FSH) are generally also tested on two occasions, approximately four to six weeks apart, and if the levels are high you are considered to have had a premature menopause.

# Can I still get pregnant?

*"My second thought was, can I have a baby?"*

Diane, 36

Whether or not the ovaries are still functioning enough to achieve pregnancy can depend on the cause. Your doctor will be able to refer you to your local gynaecology and fertility services for investigation and treatment if possible. There is no easy answer here: if there are no eggs left then you can't ovulate; yet if there are eggs, but the ovaries have stopped working for some reason, known or unknown, sometimes they suddenly start working again. In fact, one in 10 women with premature ovarian insufficiency will become pregnant, as the ovaries sporadically start to work. This means that if you want to avoid getting pregnant, you still need to use contraception.

There is a test for ovarian reserve (how much functioning ovarian tissue you may have left) which involves measuring the level of anti-mullerian hormone (AMH), which specialist doctors may request as part of the investigations. Levels of AMH don't fluctuate in the same way that FSH levels do, they peak in the mid 20s and then gradually decline; the higher the level, the more functioning ovarian tissue you have. An AMH level is not good at predicting when a menopause is going to occur, but it can be useful to help predict how successful any fertility treatment could be.

*"The news that my ovaries had stopped working at 34 was devastating, I had just found a partner and we desperately wanted to try for a baby. We thought it was game over and stopped using contraception. Well lo and behold, my boy is six now!"*

Anna, 41

*"My partner had surgery for cervical cancer which meant she couldn't get pregnant. We were considering surrogacy, so the news that I was going through a premature menopause was devastating. I felt it was my fault, my ovaries didn't work, it was me. It took us a long time to consider other options but now we have two adorable children who we adopted. I am so grateful for them."*

Jo, 42

## Now what?

Depending on the cause, you are likely to be offered hormone replacement therapy (HRT). While many women have concerns about the risks vs the benefits of HRT (discussed more in chapters 11, 12 and 13), it is important to remember that in premature menopause we are simply replacing the hormones which would normally be present anyway until, on average, age 51, so any potential risks do not apply at an earlier age. In fact, the HRT is not just to control your symptoms, but to protect your health and decrease your risk of osteoporosis and cardiovascular disease, so the risk is actually in not taking it! HRT always involves oestrogen; if you still have your uterus then it will also involve progesterone and some women will also need testosterone.

If you have had surgery or medication which has induced the menopause, the hormonal change and therefore the symptoms are very sudden. If this is the case you may need higher levels of oestrogen to control your symptoms.

But you may still need contraception, as mentioned above, and so an alternative to HRT is to use the combined oral contraceptive pill, thereby replacing the required oestrogen at the same time as providing contraception. The hormones in the combined pill will act as the hormone replacement therapy, though they are at a higher dose than in HRT. There are some concerns about the drop in hormone level in the traditional "pill-free week" at the end of a pack of pills, but you don't have to have a break between the packs (called "tailored pill-taking"; please discuss with your GP). As long as there are no other risk factors, the combined contraceptive pill can be used until the age of 50 and then you can change to HRT. Alternatively, if you have a risk factor which means you can't use the combined pill, you could have a progesterone hormone coil (an intrauterine system – IUS) for both contraception and womb protection, and then oestrogen – either via patch or gel through the skin, or orally – for your oestrogen replacement.

HRT is generally used at least until the early 50s (at least age 51), the same as the average person going through the menopause, though of course, if you are symptomatic you can use it for longer.

So there are options, whether or not you require contraception and whether or not you wish to have a regular withdrawal bleed, or no bleeds at all, whichever suits you best.

If you have a genetic condition which means that you never had periods, you may not develop symptoms related to declining hormone levels. If your hormone levels have always been low, you may not notice any change. But this doesn't mean that you don't need treatment – you will still be offered HRT until your early 50s to protect your bones and cardiovascular health.

## Combined oral contraceptive pill or HRT?

Both HRT and the combined oral contraceptive pill contain oestrogen and progesterone. Either can be used to treat symptoms and decrease the risk of conditions such as osteoporosis. However, HRT can contain body-identical hormones, while the combined oral contraceptive pill contains synthetic versions. Body-identical HRT has fewer risks than the combined pill but will not provide contraception, which may still be needed. It is also important to note that the combined oral contraceptive pill may not always be suitable, for example if you have migraines with aura, or if you are over the age of 35 and smoke. In this case, HRT may be offered, perhaps with the Mirena coil to act as both the progesterone component and as contraception. Note that the combined pill is contraindicated over the age of 50; the discussion in this paragraph refers to the situation of a premature menopause.

# Are there any consequences of having an early menopause?

*"I felt less of a woman."*

Helen, now 44

Aside from menopausal symptoms, there can be a huge psychological burden with being diagnosed with premature ovarian insufficiency, with feelings of loss and failure being very common. And if you add in struggles with fertility issues, these feelings can become overwhelming. Please see your doctor for help. There are various treatments available – both medication and psychological therapies – as well as support groups. The Daisy Network is the UK premature ovarian insufficiency charity and has lots of information and support available (www.daisynetwork.org).

In Chapter 9, the later medical consequences of the menopause are discussed such as osteoporosis and an increased risk of cardiovascular disease. The earlier you experience the menopause the higher your risk of developing these conditions which is why HRT or hormones in the form of the combined contraceptive pill are offered. Without HRT there is an 80% increase in coronary heart disease deaths in women who have a menopause under the age of 40, when compared to women who have it between 49 and 55. You may be offered a bone density scan (DEXA) to assess your bones and need for treatment, and these may be repeated approximately every two years or so thereafter. It is advised that you have a diet rich in calcium and vitamin D, or you may be advised take a supplement containing 1,000 mg of calcium and 800 IU of vitamin D per day to further decrease your osteoporosis risk.

*"Now my friends are all having symptoms like flushes and sweats I have become the guru, especially about HRT. I am now symptom-free!"*

Francesca, 50, had her last period aged 37

## Menopause due to cancer

The combination of cancer and the menopause can be difficult. Treatments for cancer, be they surgery, chemotherapy or radiotherapy, can lead to a premature menopause. In addition, hormone treatments for certain breast cancers can be given for a period of years after cancer treatment. Depending on the medication used, these either block or stop the production of oestrogen in the body. Medical or surgical menopause may lead to more severe symptoms than a non-induced menopause, due to the sudden drop in the levels of hormones.

Whether or not your cancer treatment will induce a premature menopause will depend on the type of cancer and its treatment, as well as on other factors such as your age. An induced menopause may be either temporary or permanent. For instance, while surgical removal of the ovaries is permanent, the impact of radiotherapy or chemotherapy can be either permanent or temporary. This seems to be related to age and how close you are to a natural menopause. It is more likely that an induced menopause will be temporary if you undergo chemotherapy or radiotherapy in your 20s than in your 40s.

## What perimenopause/menopause treatments are available after a cancer diagnosis?

The available treatments will depend on the type of cancer you had and what, if any, treatment you continue to receive. If you had a non-hormone-dependent cancer, for example bowel cancer, then you can take HRT and indeed this will decrease your risk of other conditions such as osteoporosis. If you have had a hormone-dependent cancer, then you may be offered alternatives to HRT for symptom control, you may be referred to a menopause clinic, or you can discuss the issue with your oncologist. Depending on the individual risks and benefits, HRT is sometimes still prescribed. Other non-hormonal treatments are available and can be used, regardless of whether you had a hormone-dependent cancer. For more information, please see chapter 14.

### SUMMARY POINTS

- Premature menopause is defined as menopause before the age of 40.
- It can be caused by medication such as chemotherapy, or surgery, infection or other causes.
- It is treated with HRT until at least the average age of menopause in order to maintain bone and cardiovascular health.
- Depending on the cause, contraception may still be required.

# Part Two

# THE MENOPAUSE AND ME

# CHAPTER 4:

# THE HEAT IS ON

———◆———

*"I was in the middle of a presentation at work, it was going OK, I wasn't nervous as it is part of my job and I was in a room of colleagues. And then it came over me like a wave, a wall of heat like I had just entered a sauna. I could feel my face going bright red and the sweat dripping off me, my blouse going patchy and my colleagues looking at me in alarm. My first hot flush."*

Sandy, 43

There are many symptoms relating to the menopause, both physical and psychological, and they may strike when you are younger than you expect. After all, as discussed earlier, the perimenopause describes the time from when you start to get symptoms until after your last period so you can be symptomatic years before your periods stop. Alternatively, you may not notice symptoms until after your periods stop. And those symptoms can go on for far longer than you may have thought. Generally, symptoms start in the few months or years before the menopause, on average at around 45, though they can start about ten years earlier. After the menopause, symptoms last four years on average, but can persist for around a decade.

The symptoms are due to the lower levels of oestrogen in the body. Oestrogen doesn't just affect the ovaries – there are oestrogen receptors everywhere, in your breasts, your skin, your brain – so the symptoms can be wide ranging. About four out of five women will have symptoms related to the menopause, and of those affected some women will find their symptoms significantly worse and more debilitating than others, with about one in four women who experience symptoms being severely affected by them.

This chapter deals with many of the common symptoms you may be experiencing. (Menstrual changes are covered separately in Chapter 6, loss of libido and other sex-related changes are covered in Chapter 7 and urinary symptoms in Chapter 5.) The purpose of this list isn't to depress you; rather, it is to reassure you that you are not alone. You may also find there are symptoms on this list that you have been experiencing and hadn't realized are related to the menopause – in which case it will help you to consider getting help and treatment. It's not a checklist and you don't need to get a full set; you may have one symptom and not others. And remember: you can still get help even if you are still having your periods!

It is also important to note that cultures from around the world may experience different symptoms, or may use various forms of language to express those symptoms. For example, women from Afro-Caribbean backgrounds are likely to experience hot flushes for longer periods of time, women from Japan are more likely to complain of fatigue, and women from South Asia are more likely to describe body pains.

# How many symptoms of the perimenopause and menopause are there?

Lots.

It is often quoted that there are 34 separate symptoms of the perimenopause and menopause. Others suggest 50, 66 or even as many as 100! Potentially, the number varies because some symptoms overlap and some lists group these together. The more common symptoms such as hot flushes or sweats are the best known, but for many women they are not the only signs. In fact, when I list symptoms to my patients, women often start nodding along and are surprised at how many can be attributed to the perimenopause and menopause.

Symptom lists and checkers are useful because they can help you to notice issues affecting your whole body and can help you to keep track. Perhaps you will notice a difference after making a lifestyle change or starting medication, or you may notice something getting worse over a few years. As some of the symptoms can be vague, it may be difficult to pinpoint exactly when they started or even to piece them together to get the whole picture. Getting to know your body, what is normal for you and what is changing, can be empowering. It is also a useful tool for your doctor!

The symptom tracker below is divided into sections: physical health, psychological health and genitourinary health (meaning genital and urinary organs) as a subdivision of physical health. Symptoms that can have both physical and psychological causes (e.g. insomnia) are repeated across sections. The simplest method is to tick the yes or no box for each symptom, having thought back over the last month, or perhaps three months. You can go into more detail and put ticks in the boxes for how often/the extent to which each symptom has been bothering you – a little, a medium amount (perhaps on half the days), or a lot – maybe nearly every day. There is also a section for you to write comments.

| Symptoms | No | Yes – affects me a little | Yes – affects me a medium amount | Yes – affects me a lot | Comments |
|---|---|---|---|---|---|
| **Physical symptoms** | | | | | |
| Hot flushes | | | | | |
| Sweats/night sweats | | | | | |
| Palpitations (feeling your heart beating quickly/ irregularly/ strongly) | | | | | |
| Insomnia (difficulty sleeping) | | | | | |
| Headaches | | | | | |
| Muscle and joint aches/pains | | | | | |
| Fatigue – lack of energy | | | | | |
| Tinnitus (hearing a noise such as a ringing or buzzing in the ears when no external sound is present) | | | | | |

| Symptoms | No | Yes (a little) | Yes (medium) | Yes (a lot) | Comments |
|---|---|---|---|---|---|
| Dizziness/feeling faint | | | | | |
| Pins and needles/ lightning pains/ electric shock sensation in any part of the body | | | | | |
| Shortness of breath/breathing difficulties | | | | | |
| Loss of libido (loss of interest in sex) | | | | | |
| Changes to periods – may become heavier/lighter/ irregular/more frequent | | | | | |
| Tender breasts | | | | | |
| Lumpy breasts (breast changes always need to be assessed by a healthcare professional) | | | | | |
| Dry/itchy skin (formication) | | | | | |
| Oral health changes – e.g. change in taste; dry mouth; burning mouth syndrome; inflamed, bleeding, painful gums; loose teeth | | | | | |

| Symptoms | No | Yes (a little) | Yes (medium) | Yes (a lot) | Comments |
|---|---|---|---|---|---|
| Cold flushes | | | | | |
| Restless legs | | | | | |
| Change to or increased body odour | | | | | |
| Increased food sensitivities | | | | | |
| Increased allergies | | | | | |
| Digestive issues – e.g. bloating, cramping, abdominal pain, constipation, diarrhoea, indigestion, heartburn | | | | | |
| Weight gain | | | | | |
| Thinning hair | | | | | |
| | | | | | |
| **Genitourinary symptoms** | | | | | |
| Vulval/vaginal dryness | | | | | |
| Vulval/vaginal irritation/pain/ soreness/burning | | | | | |

| Symptoms | No | Yes (a little) | Yes (medium) | Yes (a lot) | Comments |
|---|---|---|---|---|---|
| Painful sex | | | | | |
| Painful episiotomy scar | | | | | |
| Shrinking of the labia/clitoris | | | | | |
| Genital skin thinning/splitting | | | | | |
| Bleeding after sex (always needs to be assessed by a healthcare professional) | | | | | |
| Painful cervical screening (smear test) | | | | | |
| Recurrent urinary tract infections | | | | | |
| Urge urinary incontinence (needing to pass urine urgently) | | | | | |
| Stress urinary incontinence (incontinence on coughing/ sneezing/jumping etc.) | | | | | |
| Pelvic organ prolapse | | | | | |

| Symptoms | No | Yes (a little) | Yes (medium) | Yes (a lot) | Comments |
|---|---|---|---|---|---|
| **Psychological symptoms (mind/mood symptoms)** | | | | | |
| Anxiety | | | | | |
| Low mood | | | | | |
| Depression | | | | | |
| Irritability (mood swings) | | | | | |
| Panic attacks | | | | | |
| Brain fog | | | | | |
| Difficulty concentrating | | | | | |
| Memory problems | | | | | |
| Fatigue | | | | | |
| Insomnia (difficulty sleeping) | | | | | |
| Loss of libido (loss of interest in sex) | | | | | |
| Loss of pleasure in things | | | | | |
| Low or reduced self-esteem/loss of confidence | | | | | |

# PHYSICAL SYMPTOMS

———◆———

## Vasomotor symptoms – hot flushes (flashes) and sweats

Up and down the country, whatever the weather may be there is a war raging and the battle lines are clear. I know this because my patients tell me about it! Women in their 20s and 30s are turning up the heating as they are cold, but from their 40s upwards they are turning the heating off and hanging out the window, while their partners are turning it back on and a row ensues! While you may have heard of yo-yo dieting, this is the yo-yo heating dance – one turns it down, the other turns it up. And sleeping next to a boiling, heat-radiating partner is no longer the comfort it once was. Add in a heatwave and it can be torture.

This is the classic menopausal symptom, and indeed the commonest, affecting three or four out of every five women. For some, they are few and far between, but for about one in five women they are frequent and so severe they can be disabling, affecting sleep, relationships, work and life in general. And they can go on and on, on average for about two years but in some cases for as long as 10–15 years!

Hot flushes generally last about 3–5 minutes, but they can last longer (up to about 30 minutes) and can occur multiple times a day. A flush starts as an uncomfortably warm and then hot feeling, often in the chest and the face. Although you may feel very hot this may not be visible in your face, though you may blush and some women do go red.

A hot flush is often accompanied by sweating, sometimes just on the forehead and hands, but it can be worse, affecting the whole body. Sweating over the whole body can also happen at night – women describe waking up, literally drenched in sweat, soaking their nightclothes or sheets. Along with a flush you may experience palpitations, dizziness, anxiety or a headache.

What mustn't be underestimated here is how severe these can be for some women, who experience multiple debilitating and often embarrassing sweats per day, affecting their lives, relationships and work. This is more than feeling a bit hot!

## Why?

Humans can only survive when our bodies are at what is actually quite a small range of temperatures. Whatever the weather conditions outside we have to control our body temperature; too cold and we become hypothermic (our core body temperature drops too low), which can be fatal. Too hot can be just as dangerous – think how you feel with a fever, and that is only a couple of degrees Celsius higher than normal. So the rather sophisticated thermoregulatory centre in our brains works to keep us in the desired range, making us sweat when we are hot, or shiver if cold. Sensitive as this centre is, it doesn't respond to changes within about half a degree Celsius (known as the null zone), otherwise we would bounce between sweating and shivering all the time. Which we don't. Except during the perimenopause, when the body seems to respond to tiny changes, something as small as moving rooms or having a hot drink, or maybe even changes which aren't there. The thermoregulatory centre seems to stop working properly.

We aren't exactly sure why this happens, but it is thought that the changing levels of oestrogen affect the production of chemicals in the brain such as serotonin and noradrenaline which then seem to disrupt the working of the thermoregulatory centre, resulting in your hot flushes and sweats. And yet it can't just be that, as some women continue to get flushes years after their last period, when the levels of oestrogen have settled at their new lower level, so perhaps there has been a change to the thermoregulatory centre itself and not just how it responds to various neurotransmitters.

When your brain thinks that the body temperature is rising, it tries to counteract this to bring the temperature down, resulting in the hot flush and sweats. The brain sends messages to widen or dilate the blood vessels near the skin with the aim of cooling the blood as it passes through the skin to cool you down. Sweating is one of the body's methods of cooling down, so if your brain thinks it is too hot it will signal your body to start sweating.

## What can I do?

There are various lifestyle factors which can cause or worsen flushes:

- Being overweight.
- Smoking.
- Drinking too much caffeine.
- Eating spicy foods or foods containing monosodium glutamate.

For more information on how a healthy lifestyle can help with menopausal symptoms, please see pages 111-119.

HRT is effective in managing hot flush and night-sweat symptoms. For more information, see chapters 11, 12 and 13.

Other medical treatments that may be prescribed include clonidine (see page 291); antidepressants such as SSRIs, in particular paroxetine (see page 293); or SNRIs, in particular venlafaxine (see page 295); or other medications such as gabapentin, pregabalin (see page 297); and cognitive behavioural therapy (see page 298) – see the relevant page references for full details of these medications' usage, side effects and contraindications in Chapter 14.

Certain medications can also cause flushes (for example calcium channel blockers such as amlodipine, which can be used to treat high blood pressure), so it is worth checking with your pharmacist or GP if a medication could be making things worse.

What you wear can also help:

◆ Layer up. Wearing lots of thin layers of clothing instead of one thick one can be useful as you can take off or add back on as needed.

◆ Avoid man-made fibres such as nylon or polyester and stick to natural fibres such as cotton, linen or viscose (sorry about the increased ironing – you could just ignore it). Man-made fibres are not breathable, so the sweat gets trapped instead of being absorbed or evaporating so you feel clammy much earlier.

The following can help with the night sweats:

◆ Swap to a lower tog duvet (or even two single duvets if your partner is still cold).

◆ Use cotton sheets instead of polycotton or man-made fibres.

- Try to keep your bedroom cool – leave windows or doors open, or try a fan.
- Inserting cooling gel pads onto your pillow can help as they keep your pillow cool to rest your hot head on!
- You can even get larger cooling gel mats for your bed, so you have something cool to lie on.
- Pop your bedding in the freezer.

# Insomnia

*"I just can't sleep, if only I could sleep I think I could manage everything else. But I can't and the more I can't the more that I worry I can't and then won't be able to manage the next day, which then of course I don't as I haven't slept."*

Helen, 48

*"I am a horrible person without sleep and I feel horrible as well. I will try anything to help."*

Nicole, 54

Insomnia means an inability to sleep and has affected most of us at some point in our lives. We can't get off to sleep, we wake too early and can't get back to sleep, we wake in the middle of the night multiple times and struggle each time to sleep again or we just have disturbed sleep.

Unfortunately, insomnia doesn't just affect us at night; the effects of tossing and turning all night have an impact on our days as well.

Poor or limited sleep leads to fatigue and the feeling of being in a permanent state of tiredness and exhaustion. This can then affect your mood, make you irritable, affect your concentration (which can impact you at home or at work) or even make you more likely to reach for the biscuit tin. For more information on fatigue please see page 107.

## Why?

Insomnia can have many causes, often both physical and psychological. For example, you can't sleep if you are in pain, or if you need to go to the toilet, but also if you are depressed or anxious. Likewise, in the perimenopause physical and psychological factors come into play. Progesterone is sometimes considered a sleep hormone as high levels of it can cause sleepiness by increasing the levels of a neurotransmitter (a chemical in the brain) called GABA. Therefore it would make sense that lower levels could cause insomnia, also by affecting the levels of chemicals in the brain. Add to this physical symptoms such as night sweats, joint aches and pains, as well as increasing anxiety, low mood and racing thoughts, and insomnia is very common in the perimenopause.

## What can I do?

HRT is effective in managing insomnia symptoms (for more information, see chapters 11, 12 and 13).

Sleeping pills are not the answer here; they are addictive, they stop being effective pretty quickly, requiring higher and higher doses, and they can have side effects and interact with other medications. So your doctor is unlikely to prescribe them. Over-the-counter herbal sleep remedies are available, as are non-herbal sleep medications, which generally contain a sedating antihistamine. Please do check with your pharmacist that they won't interact with any medication you are taking.

Check with your pharmacist or doctor about any medication you are taking for other reasons, as some medications can actually cause insomnia. There may be alternatives available.

If there is a physical cause stopping you sleeping – for example pain, or getting up 20 times a night to go to the toilet, or sweats and flushes – then see your doctor, as treating those symptoms may well improve your sleep. Use the tips on page 65 to help with night sweats and flushes.

Cognitive behavioural therapy (CBT) is a proven, effective treatment for insomnia. Many people struggle to sleep because their brains are still whirring away, and CBT can help with this. There are CBT-based apps available which are effective, for example the Sleepio app.

## Sleep hygiene

Sleep hygiene is very important and can help to treat insomnia. Essentially it involves creating a healthy sleep routine and environment, just as you may have done if you had babies, with a bath and a story before bed to help show them sleep was on its way. As adults, though, this routine goes out the window and we give our bodies all kinds of conflicting signals about sleep. We live in a world that is always busy and full of lights, noise and stimulation and we have to turn off the noise in order to quiet our minds and relax our bodies to prepare for sleep. Answering work emails at 11 p.m. is not conducive to this process!

◆ Think about the physical environment of your bedroom. Do you have a comfortable bed and pillows? Is the room too hot or too cold? It is too light or too noisy? If the answer is yes to any of those questions then what could help? For example, wearing ear plugs to block out noise.

◆ Make your bedroom a sanctuary of sleep, using your bed only for sleep and sex. If possible, don't use your bed for working, watching TV, using your laptop. This will help train your mind to know that getting into bed equals going to sleep.

◆ Sleep cycles are affected by exposure to light, which is why we encourage getting exposure to natural light during the day. It also means that it helps to be in darkness at night, so use thick curtains/blinds to cut out light, or alternatively try a blackout sleep mask. This is because your body notices the contrast of light in the day to increasing darkness at night, leading to the production of the hormone melatonin which plays a role in sleep.

◆ Avoid screen time – be it the television, your phone, your tablet – for at least an hour before bedtime. The blue light from the screens disrupts your sleep pattern by sending signals to the brain suggesting that it is still light and therefore must still be daytime, so does not turn on the melatonin production.

◆ Keep your phones and screens outside the bedroom, even if they are off, as you will still have an awareness that they are there. If they are on the lights and noises are disturbing, but even on silent there is an urge to check them! Keeping them outside the bedroom also means that checking your phone is not the first thing you do in the morning!

- Go to bed when you are tired. Possibly the most obvious statement, but actually many people are trying to sleep out of routine, or have stayed up late/gone out and then try to go straight to sleep. A period of relaxation and then going to bed when you feel sleepy will help.

- This one is a biggie – you need to get up at approximately the same time every day, including the weekends. Having a big lie-in at the weekend means that it is more difficult to get to sleep the next night, so you then sleep even later the next day, and the cycle gets worse and worse. So if you wake at 7 a.m. in the week, wake at around the same time at the weekend. You don't necessarily need to then rush around starting your day – you can rest and relax but not in bed asleep! This is a key point to sleep hygiene, though perhaps one of the most difficult to do, as the urge to catch up on sleep is a big one, but it actually makes the situation worse!

- Create a relaxing bedtime routine before trying to sleep, as in time this will become a trigger, reminding your mind that it is time to go to sleep. For example, you could try to get into the habit of taking a warm bath (though it is actually cooling down after the bath which helps you sleep and not the heat of the bath itself), making a warm (non-caffeinated) drink or reading a book, or any other relaxing activity.

- Exercise. There is good evidence that regular exercise, especially exercise done outside with exposure to natural daylight, can help with insomnia. However, don't exercise too late – the natural

highs from the endorphins released during exercise can stop you
sleeping, so avoid exercising for at least four hours before bedtime.

◆ Avoid caffeine, which is covered in more detail on page 115, but
avoid for at least 5–6 hours before going to bed, for example
from 5 p.m, or even earlier, after lunchtime.

◆ Avoid other stimulants, such as alcohol and smoking, in the
evening, or even better for the same time period as for caffeine.
You may feel sleepy with alcohol but although it may help you
get to sleep more quickly, it then causes disrupted sleep through
the night.

◆ Avoid eating heavy meals too late at night as these may cause
heartburn or reflux, which could again lead to insomnia.

◆ Avoid napping if possible as this means that you won't feel
tired when it is time to sleep later. If you really cannot manage
without a nap then limit it to 30 minutes before about 3 p.m. in
the afternoon.

*"I didn't think it would work, I haven't slept properly in years and it had only
been getting worse, but a few simple changes to my routine and I am sleeping
better than ever, I think!"*

Polly, 52

## What to do when you can't sleep

Stop checking the clock. Turn it around or put it somewhere out
of sight as obsessively checking the time – how many hours you
have been awake, how little sleep you are going to have – increases
your anxiety around sleep and therefore makes it harder to go
to sleep!

If you feel you have been in bed for about 30 minutes or so and haven't slept then get up, go to another room, read a book, or do another gentle activity – no screens please – and then try again when you feel sleepy. The purpose of this is to try to break the anxiety about insomnia leading to an insomnia cycle, but also to ensure that you associate your bedroom and bed with sleeping and not with lying there awake tossing and turning.

Try some of the following techniques.

### Relaxation techniques

Relaxation techniques, from the breathing techniques described opposite, meditation, mindfulness and more, are a skill, and like any skill have to be learned and the learning takes time. They are not a quick fix and it can take a few months to begin to really see a result. The techniques can help with insomnia but are also useful in dealing with hot flushes and anxiety. There are lots of different techniques and various mindfulness apps such as Headspace and Calm that can help guide you through the process. It can be useful to practise these techniques in a calm environment, perhaps lying on your bed or the couch, but in time you can practise them in different environments, which then means that you can use them in a variety of different situations.

Try this simple relaxation exercise:

◆ Focus on your breathing. Place your hands on your tummy and you should feel your hands rise as you inhale, and then fall again as you exhale. Even this step can take practice as when we are anxious we start breathing from the chest, pulling in our tummies as we breathe, when actually if you use your diaphragm to breathe your tummy should rise up with each breath. Most of us have never really thought about breathing before, it just keeps happening on its own, inhale, exhale, but focusing on the breath is the first step to many relaxation techniques.

◆ Slow your breathing down. You may find slowly counting each breath, a count to three or four for every inhalation and again for every exhalation.

◆ In your mind, scan down your body and notice any areas where there is some tension and try to focus on relaxing that area, all the time continuing your slow breathing.

◆ An alternative is to imagine a sensation of warmth, or visualize a warm light travelling through each part of your body in turn.

## 5–4–3–2–1 technique

You can add this to the simple exercise above, or use this alone with slow calm breathing in any stressful situation.

◆ 5 – Notice **five** things you can see around you, these can be objects or even spots on the ceiling or shadows.

◆ 4 – Focus on **four** things that you can touch or feel, such as the sensation of the chair or ground under you, the feel of your breath as you breathe etc.

◆ 3 – Acknowledge **three** things you can hear, like the traffic outside, the noise of your breathing or your tummy rumbling; whatever you notice!

◆ 2 – Be aware of **two** things you can smell, for example the smell from cooking dinner, or from your sheets, or of fresh air.

◆ 1 – Think of **one** thing you can taste. Is there a lingering taste in your mouth, your last cup of coffee, your toothpaste?

The purpose of this technique is not to focus on each sensation, not to become distracted by what you notice but to become more aware of your body. So if you notice a crack in the ceiling as part of five things you can see, don't focus on the whys and what to do next about the crack, simply notice it and then move on.

With any relaxation technique you may notice that unwanted thoughts or worries pop into your head. That is fine, but the aim is to not engage with them. Instead simply acknowledge that your mind has wandered off in another direction and pull your focus back to your breathing. As mentioned above, these techniques take work and practice – do them daily!

*"I started some guided relaxation techniques to help me sleep and deal with stress but actually they are really useful in other situations, when you feel anxious or annoyed. I taught my kids and we now practise together."*

Tania, 53

# Palpitations

*"I thought something must be terribly wrong, I could literally feel my heart thumping in my chest, I had never felt it before, was this a heart attack?"*

Imogen, 50

Palpitations are an awareness of your heart beat, which can be faster than normal or at its normal rate, or you may be aware that it seems to be in an unusual rhythm or skips a beat.

## Why?

Palpitations related to the perimenopause are a result of declining oestrogen and progesterone levels. They can also be linked to hot flushes or with anxiety or stress.

There are many causes of palpitations apart from the menopause, such as anaemia or thyroid issues, so please do go and see your doctor to be checked out. If you have palpitations which last longer than 5 minutes or are associated with dizziness, shortness of breath or chest pain please seek urgent medical advice.

## What can I do?

HRT is effective in managing palpitation symptoms (for more information, see chapters 11, 12 and 13).

Medical treatments and alternative remedies are covered in chapters 14 and 15, but even if you are not using HRT or other treatments there are medications which can help with palpitations perhaps related to anxiety in the perimenopause, for example a beta blocker.

There are various factors which can make palpitations worse or more frequent so avoiding these can be useful:

◆ Smoking.
◆ Alcohol.
◆ Caffeine.
◆ Monosodium glutamate (MSG, found in some Chinese food and processed foods and meats).
◆ Medications such as ephedrine or pseudoephedrine which are found in nasal decongestant sprays and cold remedies.

# Joint pain

Many women seem to put joint pain and general aches and pains down to age or lack of fitness, but in fact this symptom can also be related to the menopause.

It is common to have joint aches and pains during the perimenopause, as well as joint and muscle stiffness. These commonly affect the neck, shoulders, elbows, wrists and knees, but can be anywhere. Often it is general muscle stiffness and aches and pains, worse in the morning and easing across the day, or increased pain on exercising.

## Why?

Oestrogen is involved in lubricating the joints and it is thought that it may act as an anti-inflammatory. As levels fall, the joints can become inflamed, making them painful and feeling stiff.

## What can I do?

HRT can be effective in managing joint pain symptoms (for more information, see chapters 11, 12 and 13).

See your doctor to rule out other causes. Some women are incorrectly diagnosed with arthritis around the time of the menopause as the signs and symptoms can be similar.

◆ Don't stop exercising as this can make other symptoms worse. Exercise keeps you healthy, your joints flexible and is good for your mental health.

◆ Avoid exercise that puts a lot of stress on the joints if they are painful, for example avoid running if your knees are swollen and painful. Try a non-weight-bearing aerobic exercise such as swimming.

◆ As long as they don't interact with other medications or conditions, an over-the-counter medication like paracetamol, or an ibuprofen gel, can be helpful to relieve pain, as can ice packs.

*"I felt I could manage the odd uncomfortable night or an occasional hot flush, but the aches and pains really got me down, I just felt old."*

Georgina, 52

# Headaches

We all have experienced a headache at some point in our lives, some more frequently than others, but you may notice an increase in headaches or migraines in the perimenopause. You may have had headaches relating to ovulation or your period before, but these can increase or start during the perimenopause.

## Why?

The fluctuating levels of oestrogen and progesterone can trigger headaches and migraines. If you have migraines related to your period and your cycle length has become shorter, you will get more migraines. However, some women find that after the menopause they no longer get migraines – finally a benefit!

## What can I do?

HRT can help to manage headache symptoms (for more information, see Chapter 11) but with headaches the response to HRT is variable. If you notice a worsening in headaches on HRT please tell your doctor. Delivering the oestrogen through the skin via a patch or gel is less likely to trigger a headache.

There are various medications used for migraines, such as painkillers and a class of medication called 5-HT agonists such as sumatriptan. If you are getting regular migraines, medications can be used prophylactically to try to stop them.

- Have your eyes tested. Headaches have multiple causes, one of which is eye strain, so before you put your headaches down to the menopause get them tested!

- If you are taking over-the-counter painkillers for headaches try to watch how often you are using them as medication overuse is a common cause of headaches. Using paracetamol more than two or three times a week, or more than ten times a month for a headache can actually set off a cycle of medication overuse headache.

- If you are concerned about your headaches or if you have other neurological signs such as muscle weakness or changes in vision seek medical advice.

# Skin, hair, nails and more

## Skin changes

*"Everyone knows the really not funny joke, that if a man wants to know what his wife will look like when she gets older he should look at his mother-in-law. Only for me it is worse than that: when I look in the mirror I seem to see my father, I look like I am turning into an old man!"*

Belinda, 58

Oestrogen has many roles in the skin, including where fat is deposited, the development of collagen, and control of the pigment-producing cells of the skin. When oestrogen levels fall, you may notice any or all of the following:

### Dry skin

As the levels of oestrogen fall, the production of collagen and elastin – proteins that give the skin its strength, support and elasticity – may also decrease, and more water is lost through the skin. In the first five years after the menopause, the levels of collagen decrease in your skin by about 30%. This then slows down significantly but continues to gradually decrease. Oestrogen is also involved in stimulating the production of sebum from sebaceous glands, which keeps skin lubricated, and in the production of ceramides, which help protect the skin. This leads to thinner, less flexible-looking skin that can look dry and dehydrated and can become itchy. You may also notice that your skin takes longer to heal after the menopause.

## Itchy skin

The hormone changes of the perimenopause and menopause can also lead to the skin becoming itchy (pruritus). This may be related to the skin becoming dryer as described above, or more sensitive to products such as soaps. Parasthesia is a change in sensation to the skin, which can cause itching accompanied by tingling, prickling or even numbness. Formication can also occur, which is the sensation of insects crawling under the skin. Once itching starts it can lead to scratching, setting up the "itch-scratch cycle", where the more you scratch, the more inflamed and irritated the itchy skin becomes, which makes it more itchy, and so the cycle starts again.

## Oily skin

Oestrogen also has an anti-acne effect, which is why many women find that their skin improves when they are pregnant or on the contraceptive pill. As oestrogen levels fall it seems to unmask the effects of testosterone; and without the oestrogen to balance or counteract its effects in the skin, the testosterone can dominate. This means that the testosterone can stimulate the sebaceous glands, making them secrete thick, greasy sebum. Some women develop oily skin or adult acne as a result.

## Fine lines, wrinkles and saggy skin (oh my!)

Oestrogen plays a role in where we store fat in the body. As oestrogen levels fall, fat distribution changes, with more fat being deposited in the tummy, bottom and thighs. This means that there is less fat to support the skin in the face, neck, chest and hands, which can then become saggier and start to wrinkle. The loss of oestrogen also leads to lower amounts of supportive collagen in the skin, more fluid being lost through the skin, and less blood supply to the skin itself, all meaning that the skin becomes less elastic and flexible. This loss of elasticity leads to the formation of fine lines and wrinkles.

### Sensitivity to sun damage

Over time the skin becomes more sensitive to the sun. Less oestrogen means lower levels of collagen and elastin and so the skin is less efficient at repairing itself, particularly after damage from UV light from the sun. Oestrogen also controls the production of the skin pigment melanin; as oestrogen levels fall so does the amount of melanin being produced in the skin. Reduced melanin can result in paler skin, which is more susceptible to sun damage.

Conversely, though, in some areas of the skin the amount of melanin produced actually increases during this time, as the regulatory control of oestrogen is lost. This generally occurs in areas that are more regularly exposed to the sun, such as the face, neck, chest, arms and hands, leading to age spots or brownish-coloured patches.

---

The changes that are happening in your skin are also happening in your vulva, vagina and urinary tract. So if you notice that your skin is becoming drier, saggier and more wrinkly, the same loss of elasticity may well be happening in the vagina, urethra and bladder. For more information on these changes please see chapters 5 and 7.

---

## Why?

As ever, the declining levels of oestrogen and progesterone are to blame for the changes in your skin around the menopause and beyond. There are receptors for these hormones in the skin, and indeed all over the body, and falling levels have an impact on every tissue, including skin.

## What can I do?

◆ Use sunscreen every day, come sun, come rain, come cloud! Look for one with a minimum of SPF 30 to protect against the UVB rays from the sun and a high star rating – preferably five out of five stars – to protect against UVA rays. Check the packaging for both ratings.

◆ Moisturize! Using a good moisturizer will help keep your skin hydrated and prevent the extra water loss through the epidermis (upper layer of the skin). Your daily moisturizer or even some make-up can provide SPF protection, but just make sure that it is at least factor 30. Avoid scented moisturizers.

◆ If your skin is dry and/or itchy avoid long hot baths/showers, which can further dehydrate the skin. Washing with soap is also not advisable, especially with scented products, which can cause more irritation. Wash yourself using an over-the-counter emollient instead. Emollients can be used multiple times a day, all over the body, to put moisture back into the skin and therefore ease itching. Pat yourself dry after washing rather than rubbing, which can irritate the skin. Importantly, try not to scratch; apply a cold compress or a soothing emollient instead. If the itching is severe at night, you can try wearing gloves to minimize scratching.

◆ HRT (covered in more detail in Chapter 11) can help improve
the texture and quality of your skin by replacing oestrogen,
therefore ensuring the skin's hydration, and boosting the collagen
and other proteins in the skin. HRT is not given solely for
cosmetic reasons, but many women feel that the effects on the
skin are an added bonus!

## Nail changes

*"I knew that my periods might go haywire before they went, knew about hot
flushes and my friends told me about being irritable, but I didn't know that
so many parts of my body would be affected. It sounds like something little but
I never liked much about my appearance but I was proud of my nails. I had
good strong nails but they seemed to really weaken and break and flake all the
time. Perhaps it isn't the medical answer to it but an occasional manicure gives
me back my 'perfect' nails!"*

Beth, 56

During the perimenopause and after the menopause, you can
experience weak, dry, brittle nails that may break and flake. The
vertical ridges in the nails may also become more prominent.

### Why?

Nails are made of a protein called keratin, which is the same protein
that makes hair, even though hair and nails have totally different
textures! The falling levels of oestrogen in the body affect keratin
production and can cause nails to become more dehydrated, which
makes them weaker and more brittle.

**What can I do?**

- Ensure that you keep well hydrated and use a good moisturizer on your hands and nails. This can be done regularly, after every hand wash.
- Wear rubber gloves to do the washing-up!
- Prolonged use of false nails or gel varnishes (and the acetone needed to remove them) can further weaken nails, so you may wish to avoid them.

## Hair changes

Approximately one third of women will develop some hair loss after the menopause. The hair itself becomes thinner and there can be what is known as "male pattern" hair loss, which is loss around the crown and temples. Pubic hair and hair in the armpits also change; growth slows down and the hairs may become sparser or thinner.

*"I have always had a thick head of hair, more of it than I ever really knew what to do with. But it started falling out at an alarming rate, at the same time as unwanted hair was appearing elsewhere! I thought only men went bald – is it going to happen to me?"*

Eve, 60

*"Perhaps it shouldn't matter but it does, much of who I think I am, my femininity and womanhood is wrapped up in my hair. So when I began to find fistfuls of hair in the shower at the same time as my periods getting further and further apart I felt that I was less of a woman."*

Amelie, 58

Hair loss around the menopause is often at the front of the head, around the hairline of the temples and forehead, and at the top of the head, but more generalized thinning of the hair can occur.

Facial hair may begin to appear, particularly on the upper lip, chin or peach fuzz around the cheeks.

*"I remember hours of painful electrolysis when I was younger but I got rid of the dark hair on my upper lip. Now my moustache is growing back and even more frighteningly it is being joined by what seems to be a hairy chin!"*

Carole, 62

## Why?

Every hair goes through various phases including a growing and resting phase before falling out. Oestrogen plays a role in keeping hair in the growing phase so the declining levels of the hormone will affect hair growth. Reduced oestrogen levels mean that hair spends less time in the growing phase, so it cannot grow as long as previously before falling out. Lower oestrogen levels also mean that the effects of testosterone are no longer countered by oestrogen, and testosterone can also encourage hair loss.

There can be multiple causes of hair loss so it may be worth seeing your doctor. For example, low iron levels from heavy periods (which are more common in the perimenopause) will also lead to hair loss, and this can be mitigated with treatment to bring the iron levels back up.

Decreasing levels of oestrogen mean that there isn't enough to counteract the effects of testosterone, which can lead to the appearance of facial hair.

**What can I do?**

Avoid other factors that can weaken or damage hair, for example hair dyes, excessive heat application such as hair straighteners, or pulling your hair into very tight hairstyles, like braids.

As for facial hair, there are various methods of removal if you desire: permanent hair removal using lasers is available. This is most effective when the hair contains pigment and is darker than the colour of your skin, so it is less likely to work on white or blonde hairs. Electrolysis is another method of hair removal that can be permanent (with repetitive treatments) and works on all hair and skin colours. Non-permanent methods such as waxing are also available, along with threading or tweezing.

# Weight gain

*"Like a lot of people I have always yo-yoed up and down a bit with my weight. But once I hit my mid forties the yo-yo seemed to get stuck at up, it just got so much harder to lose weight and so much easier for it to creep on."*

Tina, 51

Many women will notice that they gain weight around the perimenopause and menopause, even though they may not have changed their diet and exercise regimes. You may also notice that your shape changes, with fat being stored on your tummy as opposed to on your hips – "middle-aged spread"!

## Why?

Weight gain and control of your weight is an extremely complicated issue and this remains true around the time of the menopause. The majority of people in the UK have a BMI over 25 (considered overweight) even before entering the perimenopause, which worsens the issue. The older we get after about age 40, the slower our basal metabolic rate (BMR) becomes. This means that even if we eat exactly the same number of calories as when we were younger, we will gain weight. In addition, the older we get, the more muscle mass we lose. Muscle works harder than fat to burn calories, even when you are resting, so the less muscle you have, the more likely you are to gain weight.

Although most of the oestrogen produced by the body comes from the ovaries, a weaker form of oestrogen is made in fat cells. As the levels of oestrogen fall, your body will try to make more, so you may find that you gain weight as the body tries to make more fat cells in order to produce oestrogen. Other symptoms can also have an impact. For example, insomnia affects the levels of hunger and satiety hormones, affecting how much you eat. Add to this joint and muscle pain, mood changes, and what can be crushing fatigue, as well as concerns about leaking urine (meaning that women may tend to exercise less than previously), then it's no wonder that weight gain can be a problem. Oestrogen affects how and where we store fat, and it is the falling oestrogen levels which mean that fat is deposited around the tummy, changing the shape of your figure.

*"How can I exercise? I hurt all over and then even when I do muster enough energy to do anything I would wet myself a bit. It isn't worth it."*

Carol, 56

## What can I do?

If only I had an easy answer to this one! Weight gain and loss is, as I said, extremely complex. The saying "eat less and move more" sounds straightforward but it doesn't mean that it is remotely easy to do. For more on healthy lifestyle measures, turn to pages 111-119.

If you have obesity, or if your weight is over a particular level together with other cardiovascular risk factors, there are weight-loss medications available on prescription. Bear in mind that these can have side effects. Weight-loss (bariatric) surgery is an effective treatment for obesity but it is only available on the NHS if your body mass index (BMI) is over 40, or between 35 and 40 if you have another condition such as type 2 diabetes, and only after other weight-loss methods have not worked. (For more on BMI, see page 111.)

However, having too low a BMI is not good for your health either. Fat cells are involved in the production of oestrogen, even after the menopause, albeit in a weaker form to that made in the ovaries pre-menopause, but some is still made. Having a particularly low body weight is not good for your bone or general health. So we are aiming to maintain a healthy weight.

There is often a concern that HRT will lead to weight gain, but there is no evidence that this is the case. In fact, if you are on HRT and therefore symptoms such as insomnia and bodily aches and pains are being tackled, you are more likely to exercise. The oestrogen component of HRT can sometimes lead to fluid retention, which is not true weight gain, but this tends to resolve itself and disappear after a few months.

*"I always had a flattish tummy, even with a curvy hourglass figure. But my figure seemed to change shape, I went from an hourglass to an apple shape, the 'flattish' tummy turned rounder and rounder!"*

Ellie, 55

# Breast changes

*"My breasts were my pride and joy, the only bit of my body that I liked. But now they have fallen down, like deflated balloons. I'm saving up to have them lifted."*

Jill, 59

Breast soreness and tenderness can occur during the perimenopause, and your breasts may even seem to change size from week to week. You may notice that they are painful or tender, particularly before your period, and/or you may notice more lumps in the breasts. After the menopause, the breasts can change shape, get smaller, sag, and become softer. You may also notice that they are lumpier than before. Always get any changes checked out by your doctor.

## Why?

The irregular ovulation of the perimenopause means that your breasts are irregularly exposed to hormones such as progesterone, which can make them sore and tender, as part of pre-menstrual syndrome. After the menopause, the fall in oestrogen affects the breast tissue itself. The glandular tissue which was involved in milk production shrinks and the breasts become mainly composed of fatty tissue.

## What can I do?

If you notice any breast changes, such as lumps or areas of thickening, please see your doctor to be checked over. For more information about breast awareness and self-examination please see page 213.

For pain:

◆ Wear a well-fitting, supportive bra. If you have never had a bra fitted before, now may be the time. Get help to ensure that your bra fits and provides the support you need.

◆ Some women report that, for tender breasts, wearing a soft bra at night helps.

◆ You can try rubbing in an over-the-counter non-steroidal anti-inflammatory pain-relieving gel such as ibuprofen gel.

◆ Please see your doctor if the pain doesn't improve.

For change in shape and firmness:

◆ Again, wear a well-fitting, supportive bra.

◆ There are no muscles in your breasts, but the breasts are held up by your pectoral muscles, so exercising these (such as by doing press-ups) can help the appearance of the breasts.

◆ Plastic surgery can involve lifting the breasts and using implants to change their appearance. This is not available on the NHS.

# Less common physical symptoms

## Tinnitus

Tinnitus is when you can hear a noise without there being any external sound. It is often a ringing or buzzing noise. Tinnitus affects approximately 10–15% of people and if severe can impact on sleep and quality of life. For some women, tinnitus starts or increases during the perimenopause and menopause.

### Why?

The exact cause of tinnitus in general is not known, though it can be related to hearing loss. Why it should occur or heighten during the perimenopause is still unknown. There are receptors for oestrogen in the ear and in the auditory neural pathways but how changing hormone levels can cause tinnitus is not yet clear.

### What can I do?

If you have tinnitus it is important to get your hearing checked as it can be associated with hearing loss. Treatment may relate to an underlying cause but there is no specific medication to treat tinnitus itself. Some people find sound helpful, having soft music or noise in the background, but avoid loud noises and stress as these can increase symptoms. Try to ensure that you are getting enough sleep. Stress management techniques such as yoga, mindfulness and deep breathing can also be helpful.

## Restless legs syndrome

Restless legs syndrome (RLS) is an uncomfortable urge to move your legs at night, often with a tingly, crawling sensation in the legs. It can appear or increase during the perimenopause and menopause.

### Why?

RLS can be due to an underlying condition such as iron deficiency anaemia. The reasons for it occurring without an underlying condition are not known, nor why it can occur or worsen in the perimenopause and menopause. It also isn't clear if RLS leads to insomnia, or if insomnia can make you more aware of restless legs. The fact that RLS is more common in women than in men, and can develop during the menopause transition, suggests that a hormonal factor may be involved.

### What can I do?

If there is a known underlying cause then this should be treated. Lifestyle measures such as avoiding stimulants (e.g. alcohol, smoking and caffeine), regular physical activity (particularly yoga) and good sleep hygiene may be helpful. Taking a warm bath before bed and massaging your legs may also help relieve RLS.

## Dizziness

The word dizziness is often used to describe feeling light-headed or unsteady, as if the room is spinning, or of having the sensation that you are going to faint.

## Why?

The cause of dizziness in the perimenopause/menopause is not fully understood. It could be related to other conditions, to hormonal changes, or there could be other reasons for it. Some theories suggest that there could be changes to the middle ear, which is involved in balance; or that the hormonal changes affect the body's response to insulin, meaning that your blood sugar levels may drop too low; or it may be related to hot flushes, migraines or fatigue. Dizziness can also occur with increased stress and anxiety, which may also be related to the menopause.

## What can I do?

There are lots of causes of dizziness so please see your doctor so that you can be fully assessed, especially if you have other symptoms such as tinnitus, hearing loss or other neurological symptoms. It is likely that they will check your blood pressure when you are sitting and then standing. The treatment will depend on the cause of the dizziness. Eat regularly to keep your blood sugar levels stable, keep up your fluid intake and try to manage stress.

## Electric shock sensations

Electric shock sensations (ESS) are often described as a fleeting electric shock, or like the sensation of a rubber band snapping or popping under the skin, which can be painful.

## Why?

The exact cause of electric shock sensations is not known, but oestrogen may be involved as it can affect the nervous and cardiovascular systems.

## What can I do?

Exercise and physical activity, eating a balanced diet and reducing or managing stress can be helpful.

## Changes to body odour

Some people will notice a change in the amount of sweat they produce and in body odour during this time. Women report sweating much more than previously, and that their sweat smells much stronger.

## Why?

Sweating is part of the body's thermoregulatory system; it helps cool you down when you are hot. During the perimenopause and menopause the brain's thermoregulatory centre seems to stop working properly, leading to hot flushes and sweats. Sweating can also increase due to anxiety and stress, which may rise during this time, often related to other symptoms. The change in hormone levels can affect the bacteria on the skin, which can then result in a change to the smell of the sweat.

## What can I do?

Managing your hot flushes can help manage sweat and body odour – please see page 64. Antiperspirants stop the production of sweat, while deodorants mask any odour, so make sure that your deodorant also contains antiperspirants. Extra-strength antiperspirants are available over the counter and some on prescription.

## Cold flushes

Hot flushes (with or without sweats) are probably the most famous of the perimenopause and menopause symptoms, but cold flushes can also happen. This occurs when you sense a sudden cold rush, or you feel as if you have entered a cold room. A cold flush tends to last a few minutes and sometimes follows a hot flush; as the hot flush fades you may feel cold and shivery – the classic "cardigan off, cardigan on, then off again"!

### Why?

Lower levels of oestrogen affect the thermoregulatory centre in the brain, meaning that it becomes extremely sensitive to even tiny changes in temperature.

### What can I do?

Although the flushes are cold rather than hot ones, the techniques and lifestyle measures to manage them are similar. Avoid caffeine and alcohol and participate in regular exercise. Wear layers of clothing so that you can add more in a cold flush, as opposed to taking off layers in a hot one. Wearing a pair of socks at night may help keep your feet warm, which could both prevent and treat a cold flush.

## Shortness of breath

Breathing difficulties might include feeling short of breath or not being able to exercise as usual, or it might be that a pre-existing lung condition (e.g. asthma) gets worse.

## Why?

The reason for shortness of breath is not fully understood, but it is possible that the changing hormone levels affect lung function. Shortness of breath is also associated with anxiety, which can also increase during this time.

## What can I do?

Get checked out by your doctor as there are lots of causes of shortness of breath that need to be assessed. Physical activity and stopping smoking can also be helpful.

# Menopause and the mouth

The menopause can affect the mouth, gums and teeth. It is thought that oral health symptoms may be as common as hot flushes, with about half of menopausal women being affected in some way.

Symptoms can include:

- Dry mouth.
- Bleeding and painful gums (gingivitis) that may look pale, bright red or purple.
- Receding gums.
- Sensation that teeth are moving or that gaps are appearing between the teeth. This is due to periodontitis, which is

related to chronic gum disease and can affect the bones supporting the teeth.

◆ Tooth loss, which may be related to periodontitis.

◆ Metallic taste in the mouth.

◆ Phantom tastes (tasting something that isn't there).

◆ Changes in taste (often with salty, sour or peppery food).

◆ Bad breath.

◆ Pain on chewing and eating.

Burning mouth syndrome can also occur, generally in combination with an extremely dry mouth. There may be the sensation that your mouth is burning or scalding, or you may notice a tingle, rather like when you've burned your tongue on something hot. This intermittent feeling tends to affect the lips, palate and tongue.

The bones all over the body become less dense after the menopause, and this includes the bones of the face and jaw. The bones of the jaw can shrink, which again increases the risks of the teeth moving or falling out.

Some symptoms of the menopause may lead to changes that then impact on your oral health. For instance, you may crave more sugary foods, which can affect your teeth, mood changes may mean that you are less likely to eat a healthy diet or to give up smoking, or you may grind your teeth (bruxism) due to menopause-related anxiety.

## Why?

The mouth has lots of oestrogen receptor cells, especially in the mucous-producing membranes that coat the mouth and in the salivary glands that make saliva. Generally, these keep the mouth moist, which helps keep it clean and sterile. As oestrogen levels decrease, less mucous and saliva may be made. This then leads to a dry mouth which in turn means that bacteria can build up. A study in 2003 from Sweden showed that postmenopausal women had less saliva and more bacteria than women on HRT. Less saliva and more bacteria can lead to gum disease, which may present as pain or bad breath, or as bleeding or receding gums.

Oestrogen is also involved in the production of collagen, which is part of your gums. As levels of oestrogen fall, less collagen may be made which can then create issues such as gum disease. The combination of less collagen and potential gum disease (related to the lack of oestrogen) can make the gums recede. This can lead to looser teeth and it increases the chance of teeth falling out or becoming crooked.

The reason for the metallic taste, or even phantom tastes in the mouth, is not fully understood. It is currently thought to be related to an issue with cells in and around the tongue and mouth which contain oestrogen receptors.

## What can I do?

Depending on the symptom, your doctor is likely to advise you to see a dentist for oral health problems. It is therefore important that both dentists and doctors are aware of the link between the menopause and oral health.

Avoid toothpastes which contain a substance called SLS, as this can further dry out the mouth. Artificial saliva sprays may help relieve some discomfort.

THE HEAT IS ON

If you have a metallic taste in the mouth, then you may find it helpful to avoid alcohol, very acidic foods, or spicy foods, though very strong flavours can sometimes mask the metallic taste. Even changing your cutlery from metal to bamboo might help.

HRT may help treat symptoms and prevent them from worsening. According to a study in 2017, people who took HRT were 44% less likely to experience severe gum disease.

Good dental hygiene is essential, as is preventative care, so ensure that you are brushing and flossing twice each day. Make sure that you arrange regular appointments to see a dental hygienist for cleaning, as well as your dentist for check-ups. Using an electric toothbrush is more effective than a manual one for removing plaque.

## Menopause and gut health

The perimenopause and menopause can also affect your gastrointestinal system (i.e. your gut). This may lead to symptoms that are similar to those of irritable bowel syndrome (IBS), or you might notice that existing gut issues become worse. Symptoms can occur intermittently or can last a few days or weeks at a time.

Symptoms include:

- Bloating.
- Stomach pain, which may feel crampy; the pain may be relieved by emptying your bowels but not always.
- Diarrhoea, constipation or "constipated diarrhoea" – the sensation of being constipated but when you do go the stool is loose.
- The feeling of incomplete emptying after you pass stool; that there is still more that could pass.

- Increased flatulence (farting) and/or burping more than usual, feelings of trapped wind, or a very noisy, rumbling, gurgling gut.
- Urgency, the feeling that you need to rush to the toilet to open your bowels.
- Indigestion and acid reflux (heartburn) can also occur.
- There may even be more likelihood of developing food intolerances or food allergies.

## Why?

Oestrogen has a role in digestion and there are oestrogen receptor cells in the gastrointestinal system. The lower levels of oestrogen can also affect other hormones that may then impact on digestion, such as cortisol. The gastrointestinal system is full of bacteria, known as the gut microbiome, which has many roles in both gut and overall health. The gut microbiome can be influenced by oestrogen. After the menopause, lower levels of oestrogen can alter the balance of the gut microbiome, which can further impact oestrogen levels. These fluctuations can affect your gut health, metabolism (potentially causing weight gain and increased risk of other conditions), mood and cognition. The section of the microbiome that can influence oestrogen levels is called the estroblome.

Other symptoms of the menopause can have a knock-on effect on the gut. For example, anxiety can increase levels of stress hormones that affect the bowels, or depression may mean that you are less active and less likely to keep to a healthy, balanced diet, making constipation more likely. Most of us have had a churning sensation in the stomach when we are nervous, and that is because the gut and the brain are connected. The gut is in fact often called the "second brain", so what impacts on one can impact on the other, and this includes the menopause.

## What can I do?

Some of the lifestyle measures and techniques used for irritable bowel syndrome (IBS) may be helpful. For example, eating smaller, more regular meals, and chewing well so that food is substantially broken down in the mouth even before it reaches the stomach, may help with bloating and gas. Being well hydrated, drinking plenty of fluids and doing some physical activity can prevent constipation; and eating mindfully and not rushing may also be effective. Avoid fizzy drinks as these can worsen bloating, and try to limit caffeine and alcohol. You may find that keeping a food diary is useful as you may discover that certain foods are harder to digest and thus lead to bloating (e.g. vegetables like broccoli and cauliflower), or that particular fruits (e.g. plums) worsen diarrhoea. A food diary may also help you to identify other triggers, such as spicy or ultra-processed foods. Ensuring that you have enough fibre in your diet is also important, as are prebiotics, which help encourage healthy bacteria in the microbiome. You may find that seeing a dietitian is useful for managing your diet and symptoms. Mindfulness and yoga practices can also be helpful, as they are known to reduce stress levels, which can then impact on the gut. Research into the many roles of the gut microbiome is still ongoing.

There are also medications that can help control symptoms, including laxatives or fibre-based bulking agents for constipation, medications to treat diarrhoea, and antispasmodic medications that relax the gut and help to prevent cramps. Symptoms may improve with HRT. Cognitive behavioural therapy (CBT) can also help you manage symptoms and reduce stress, which may be impacting on your gut health.

It is important that you see your doctor if you have any of the following: a change in bowel habit; blood in your stool or from the anus (on the paper, mixed with the toilet water, or mixed with the stool); persistent abdominal pain (more than three weeks); extreme fatigue; or unintentional weight loss – where you lose weight without trying to. We all have a bowel habit: yours might be three times per week or three times per day; both are normal. What you need to look out for is a change from *your* normal bowel routine, where, for example, you become more or less constipated, or your bowel habit was three times per week and this changes to three times per day. We can all get diarrhoea or constipation sometimes (e.g. tummy bug or from travelling), BUT if it lasts for more than three weeks then please see your doctor. Also seek medical advice if you have persistent bloating that is not related to eating. These symptoms could be related to bowel cancer, or ovarian cancer, or other conditions that need to be assessed and ruled out.

# PSYCHOLOGICAL SYMPTOMS

———◆———

*"When I started going through the change and began to feel tearful my mother told me that she was told she had empty nest syndrome, that her overwhelming sadness was because my siblings and I had left home. She wasn't offered any help or treatment and suffered for a long time. She begged me to see the doctor to see if things were different now, thankfully they are."*

Imogen, 51

The perimenopause and menopause for many women are not easy and for a long while the mental health issues and symptoms which can arise were not even discussed. The menopause unfortunately remains taboo, and many people are concerned about the stigma associated with mental health problems, and so women are often not talking about the symptoms they have. The purpose of discussing the psychological symptoms around the menopause is not to make you feel bad, or as with the physical symptoms, not to provide you with a checklist to check off; instead, it is to help you feel less alone. It is so easy to feel isolated and as if you are the only one suffering this way, but you are not the only woman to have experienced whatever symptom you have and most importantly there is help available, you just need to tell someone that you need it.

*"For me, the hardest part was admitting that something was wrong, why couldn't I manage? Everyone else seems to, but I was overwhelmed with*

*feelings of anxiety and sadness. It took a long time for me to pluck up the courage to see the doctor, but I was so glad I did."*

Harriet, 52

The symptoms can be wide ranging but often include:

## Pre-menstrual syndrome (PMS)

Just like any other symptom of the menopause, the issues can arise while you are still having your periods. Some women find that PMS symptoms, such as irritability or low mood, get worse during the perimenopause.

*"I had sort of got used to my PMS, knew when to hide away and what helped, which for me was running, but suddenly what was once a month became every three weeks which seemed to tip the balance for me."*

Natalie, 45

## Anxiety

*"It isn't that I am worried about one thing, in fact rationally I know that I haven't got anything in particular to worry about. It is more that I am worried about everything in my life and the whole world! I am constantly on red alert, as if ready to run from a bear who wants to eat me, and have panic attacks without any obvious cause. Thankfully these have stopped since I started the medication, the anxiety is still there but better and I hope the talking therapy will help."*

Tamara, 46

Symptoms of anxiety include: feeling tense, fearful or even panicky and those fears seem to be persistent and may be all-pervasive. It can also have physical symptoms such as chest pain, shortness of breath, palpitations, shaking hands, nausea, tense muscles, difficulties sleeping (such as difficulties getting to sleep or staying asleep) and feeling fidgety, like you constantly have to be on the move.

## Depression

*"It was constant, I felt like I cried all the time, anything and nothing could set me off. I felt worthless, useless and then incredibly guilty that I felt this way when nothing bad had happened to me. I stopped eating and sleeping. It has taken a while but we have found the right combination of meds for me and I am beginning to recognize myself again."*

Yvette, 52

There is a difference between feeling sad and being depressed. After all, we are all sad sometimes. In depression these feelings are more constant, overwhelming and are associated with other negative thoughts – feelings that you are worthless, useless or a failure. You can lose interest in things that previously gave you pleasure such as a hobby or seeing friends. Physical symptoms include difficulties sleeping, often waking up very early in the morning and not being able to get back to sleep, decreased appetite or overeating, decreased libido and difficulties with memory or concentration. At its worst, when depression has sucked all the pleasure out of life, thoughts about self-harm and suicide can occur. Researchers have found that almost one in ten women experience suicidal thoughts due to menopausal symptoms. Perhaps it is no coincidence that women are at the highest risk of suicide between the ages of 45 and 49: the time when most women will experience perimenopause.

If you are experiencing these sorts of thoughts, please seek urgent medical help.

## Irritability/mood swings

*"Looking back, I was a total b\*tch, to my husband, my kids, everyone, though I mostly kept it together at work. It was like I then ran out of nice and everything they did drove me insane. I was convinced it wasn't me, that they were the problem, especially my husband! It was only when my sister said to me that I seemed angry all the time that I realized something was wrong."*

Layla, 51

Irritability is when you get annoyed and irritated by everything and nothing and are unable to control your reaction to situations as you previously did, resulting in angry outbursts, an inability to control your temper or just snapping at people. You may also notice mood swings, that your mood rapidly changes from normal to feeling low, to irritable and back again.

## Difficulties with memory and concentration

Finding it hard to concentrate and to remember things during this time is sometimes called the "menopausal brain fog" as that is how it feels – like nothing is clear anymore and you can't focus on anything. This can lead to difficulties at work and at home but it can also be incredibly frustrating and anxiety-provoking.

*"I can't remember anything. By the time I get to the fridge I can't remember why I am there and my trips to the shops have multiplied as I keep forgetting things. I can't concentrate, even on something as easy as watching TV. It is so*

*disconcerting, I don't feel I am myself and am worried I have dementia, but I am only fifty-two."*

Emily, 52

# Fatigue

*"Good God I'm knackered, like I am walking through treacle most of the time. A constant, gnawing tiredness that eats away at my patience and ability to cope with anything. I long for bed, but then can't sleep. Please help!"*

Jane, 53

Tiredness is often not solely physical and the exhaustion of the perimenopause is can be caused by lots of factors – the effects of insomnia, even iron-deficiency anaemia if you are having frequent very heavy periods, as well as the fatigue that comes with anxiety and low mood.

Even if you aren't suffering from any of the psychological conditions listed above, it is common to have thoughts which may be difficult to deal with, such as no longer feeling useful, or that you have no purpose in life or work, fear of ageing, concerns about your body image. Add into the mix what can be a constant physical reminder of the perimenopause with flushes and sweats, which may make you feel out of control, and dealing with the fatigue and after-effects of insomnia, it is not surprising that many women struggle. For more information on insomnia please see page 66.

## Why?

It's the hormones again: they affect your whole body, and that includes your brain. The falling levels of oestrogen can affect the production of chemicals in the brain such as serotonin, which some call the "happiness" neurotransmitter. Serotonin is involved in mood, sleep and even appetite. There are particularly high levels of oestrogen receptors in the hippocampus, which is important for memory and emotions, so it makes sense that these can be affected. Not all women are affected in the same way or to the same degree; this may depend on the levels of these chemicals and also sensitivity of the brain receptors to them.

But it isn't as simple as hormones and neurotransmitters (not that they in themselves are simple). Added into the mix are outside factors from life – perhaps difficulties in a relationship, the changing relationship with children, dealing with ageing or unwell parents, problems at work – or a wide range of other issues.

If you have suffered with mental health problems such as anxiety or depression in the past you are more likely to find that your symptoms either reappear or worsen around the time of the menopause. Or they can appear for the first time. And if you have suffered with pre-menstrual syndrome or postnatal depression, these again increase your risk of having psychological symptoms during this time, as your brain may be more sensitive to the effects of the changing hormone levels.

Remember that every psychological symptom is on a continuum; after all, we have all felt worried or sad on occasion, it is a normal response to particular situations. If, however, these feelings become constant or all pervasive and affect your ability to function at home, in relationships, at work or even just to exist, then please seek help. And if you are thinking about hurting yourself, please do tell someone (be it a partner, friend or family member who can then support you in accessing the help that you need), or go to the doctor yourself. If you aren't sure who to talk to, or feel unable to go to the doctor, or if it is two in the morning and you need someone to talk to, then the Samaritans are available 24 hours a day, seven days a week on freephone 116 123 from the UK. In an emergency, go straight to A&E.

## What can I do?

HRT can be used to treat low mood related to the menopause (for more information, see Chapter 11).

Many women who have been diagnosed with depression in the perimenopause have been treated with antidepressants in the form of selective serotonin reuptake inhibitors (SSRIs) or serotonin and noradrenaline reuptake inhibitors (SNRIs) (see pages 293-296). However, there is no clear evidence that using these medicines in women with low mood and depression relating to the menopause is helpful UNLESS they were previously diagnosed with depression, though they are sometimes used to treat hot flushes. In fact, unless you have previously been diagnosed with depression prior to the menopause, antidepressants should not be the first line of treatment.

Psychological therapies such as cognitive behavioural therapy (CBT) are effective at treating both depression and anxiety.

## SUMMARY POINTS

◆ The symptoms related to the menopause are many and varied, and women often say that some are unexpected.

◆ Physical symptoms can include hot flushes and sweats, insomnia, palpitations, joint pains and headaches.

◆ Psychological symptoms can include PMS-type symptoms, anxiety, depression, irritability.

◆ Changes to appearance, such as changes in skin, hair and nails and weight gain, can also occur.

# HEALTHY LIFESTYLE

———◆———

The advice given in this section is general public health advice, but you, the reader, are an individual. If you have had an eating disorder or a disordered relationship with food, exercise and eating, then you may prefer to skip over this section.

## Healthy weight, healthy diet

Your body mass index (BMI) is a marker using your height and weight to work out whether or not you are at a healthy weight. To work out your body mass index go to www.nhs.uk/live-well/healthy-weight/bmi-calculator/, or divide your weight in kilograms by your height in metres squared. A healthy BMI is between 19 and 25, overweight is 25–30 and obese is over 30. It is not a perfect marker of weight and health, and indeed no perfect marker exists, but it can be used as a very broad benchmark. Waist to height ratio can also be used: measure your height and your weight, and ideally the waist circumference will be less than half your height.

If you are overweight then losing weight will have huge health benefits, from your cardiovascular health, to reducing joint aches and pains and more. Losing weight is not as simple as eating less and moving more, as obesity is related to complex issues involving various hormones; there are also psychological and socio-economic aspects. If you can, strive for slow, steady loss of 1 to 2 lb per week, aiming to lose 5–10% of your body weight, and this will lead to a significant improvement in your health. Bear in mind that weight is not synonymous with health. Irrespective of your weight, eating a balanced diet and being physically active will have benefits, both with regard to your physical and mental health.

## What should I eat?

A healthy diet is a balanced one and that includes occasional treats. No food is off limits, no food is "naughty", "bad" or a "guilty pleasure"; it is just food, without any inherent moral value. Restricting too severely is likely to be unsustainable, which means that it won't work and could lead to unhealthy attitudes towards food. Some food is more nutritionally dense than others, some is likely to fill you up and keep you full for longer, and other food may serve to bring joy and meet a social need. The key is variety, with nothing completely off limits (unless you are allergic to it), and everything in moderation.

- Aim for at least five portions of fruit and vegetables per day, preferably with more vegetables than fruit. All forms of fruit and vegetables count: fresh, frozen, canned, dried and even one juice per day.

- Increase your fibre intake. A high-fibre diet helps prevent constipation, regulate blood sugar and cholesterol, and decrease your risk of bowel cancer. In fact, a study showed that people who ate more fibre had fewer hot flushes. Eat the skins of your fruit and vegetables and add in seeds, wholegrains, nuts and pulses.

- Cut down or limit the amount of saturated fat you eat, such as red meat and cheese, swap for poultry, fish or low-fat cheese.

◆ Avoid processed or cured meats such as sausages, cold meats and bacon, or limit them as they are not only high in saturated fat but also linked to heart disease and cancers.

◆ Some fat is good. Increase the amount of healthy fats you eat, such as oily fish, nuts and avocadoes. Aim for two portions of oily fish per week, such as salmon, sardines or mackerel which are also high in omega-3 fatty acids which are good for heart health.

◆ Try to decrease the amount of salt in your diet, to help keep your blood pressure at a healthy level. It can take a little time for your palate to get used to less salt. Increasing herbs and spices can help boost the flavour instead.

◆ Avoid processed foods, which are often high in salt, fat and sugar.

◆ Spicy food can trigger hot flushes so avoiding it can be helpful.

◆ To help keep your gut microbiome happy, aim for diversity in the fruits, vegetables, nuts, seeds, wholegrains, legumes and herbs that you eat – try to aim for around 30 different plant-based foods each week. Adding probiotic foods such as yoghurt or kefir, or fermented foods like sauerkraut or kimchi, can also be helpful.

◆ Phytoestrogens are compounds found in plants that are similar, though not exactly the same, as oestrogen. Most of the research has been around a type of phytoestrogen called isoflavones, which are found in soy beans. More research needs to be done and the results of research about isoflavones have so far been mixed. One study has shown that 50 mg of isoflavones per day (approximately 2 servings) can reduce flushes. Two servings of soy-based foods is approximately 100 g soy mince, 100 g edamame beans, or 500 ml soy drinks. Tofu is also a source of low saturated fat and protein. For more information about phytoestrogens please see page 307.

- Note that consuming soy-based foods is not the same as taking a phytoestrogen supplement.

- And plan, plan, plan. Not only does this help save money but it means that you are prepared with a healthy snack when hunger strikes!

## Vitamins and supplements

- It is advised that all adults in the UK take a supplement of 10 mcg (400 IU) of vitamin D per day between October and the end of March, as most of us do not get adequate exposure to sunshine during this time to create enough vitamin D.

- If you have osteoporosis or are at greater risk of developing it you may be advised to take a supplement of calcium and/or vitamin D – please see page 205 for more information.

- Iron supplements – if you are bleeding very heavily your doctor may request a blood test to check your iron levels and advise you if supplements are required. Unless advised by a doctor, iron supplementation is not recommended.

## What should I drink?

### Water

Drink at least six to eight glasses of water per day, or 2 litres. Take a water bottle with you and keep sipping! It doesn't have to just be water though, although try to limit juice to a maximum of one glass per day as juice is high in natural sugars. Tea and coffee do count towards your fluid intake but they are slightly diuretic so make you urinate more; the amount of liquid in the drink is likely to compensate for this, however.

## Caffeinated drinks

Caffeine can trigger hot flushes so limiting your intake of tea and coffee can be helpful. It is a stimulant, so try to avoid it in the evening and late afternoon, as it can interfere with sleep, which is often an issue around the menopause. Caffeine can also make you feel irritable, worsen anxiety, cause palpitations and increase heartburn, so there are lots of reasons to cut down! If you do drink a lot of tea or coffee regularly and want to cut down, do so gradually to try to prevent headaches, which can be related to caffeine withdrawal.

## Alcohol

Just like smoking, we all know that too much alcohol is not a healthy choice, with impacts all over the body including liver disease and various cancers. Drinking alcohol can worsen many menopause symptoms such as hot flushes, urinary symptoms such as urgency, and is even associated with an increased risk of developing osteoporosis as it can affect how calcium is absorbed into your bones. Drinking alcohol is also associated with breast cancer. Women who drink three or more alcoholic drinks per week have a significantly higher risk of breast cancer than women who abstain from alcohol.

Let's start by working out how much alcohol you actually drink as many of my patients underestimate how much they really drink each week. After all, what exactly is a unit of alcohol?

One unit of alcohol is 10 ml (or 8 g) of pure 100% alcohol, which is the amount that the average person will metabolize and process in the body in approximately one hour. What this means is that the number of units that a drink contains will depend on both the strength of the alcohol and the drink's size. As an approximate guide:

- One shot of spirits = 1 unit.
- One small glass of standard-strength 12% wine (125 ml) = 1.5 units.
- One slightly bigger glass of standard-strength wine (175 ml) = 2 units.
- Large glass of wine (250 ml) = 3 units.
- Pint of beer = 2–3 units depending on strength.
- A standard 750 ml bottle of standard-strength wine = 10 units.

So I would start by measuring your wine glasses at home as they are probably much bigger than you think! Then drink as normal for a week and write down how much you consume to get a true idea of how much alcohol you are drinking. The recommended maximum number of units for both men and women is 14 units a week. If you do drink regularly aim to have at least two to three alcohol-free days per week and avoid binge drinking.

# Exercise

Studies show that women who do cardiovascular exercise regularly have fewer menopausal symptoms, in addition to the myriad of other health benefits related to exercise. These include improvements to your cardiovascular health and helping you to manage your weight, but also psychological benefits – the natural endorphins released during exercise make you feel good! Exercise has been proven to be beneficial for various mental health conditions and is also likely to help with mood changes related to the menopause. With regard to hot flushes, studies have shown that if you are fit and exercise, exercise can reduce hot flushes. However, if you were unfit before the menopause exercise may make flushes worse initially, so start slowly and gradually work your way up.

## How much exercise and which type?

- Aim for 150 minutes of moderate-intensity exercise, such as brisk walking, per week, or 75 minutes of high-intensity exercise (where you might be a bit too short of breath to talk) such as running or HIIT training.

- It can be anything that you like, and it definitely doesn't have to be something you are good at – better that it's something that you enjoy. So if you like team sports and loved netball at school find a local netball group, but if you prefer to exercise alone then do so! Aerobics, cycling, Zumba, swimming, trampolining, rowing, whatever you like!

- Aim to work hard enough that you are able to have a conversation but would not have enough breath to sing a song!

- It all adds up, just keep moving, little and often! Or a lot and often!

- In order to protect against osteoporosis, try to ensure that some of this cardiovascular exercise is weight bearing (see page 208 for more information).

- Add in two sessions of muscle-strengthening exercise; this can be done in a gym or at home using weights. Carrying your shopping bags or doing a YouTube body-weight exercise video in your living room (no equipment required!) also counts. Equipment such as resistance bands are also useful for strengthening exercises.

- Remember the importance of warming up and cooling down. Stretching and mobility exercises also help to improve and maintain flexibility. Exercises that help stability and balance can also be useful: after all, we need balance for absolutely everything, including getting up out of a chair! Exercise such as yoga and tai chi can be of benefit in many of these areas. Balance exercises can be as simple as practising standing on one leg.

- Have a think about what obstacles prevent you from exercising, or being more physically active, and about how these barriers can be removed. For example, are you put off because your breasts hurt during exercise? This may be improved with a well-fitting sports bra. Are you limited by time? Maybe shorter 10-minute bursts of exercise are more helpful than longer sessions; it still counts. Hindered by the presence of young children? They can join in too!

- As the slogan says "every little helps", so try to incorporate physical activity into your daily life: walk up the escalator or take the stairs instead of using the lift; get off the bus one stop earlier and walk; run up and down the stairs a few times at home, just keep moving!

- Pelvic floor exercises – all women need to do these, every day! For more information on how to do pelvic floor exercises correctly please see page 123.

# Smoking

Smoking is linked to respiratory diseases (such as COPD and emphysema), many forms of cancer (not just lung cancer, but cervical cancer and others) and increases your risk of cardiovascular disease such as heart attack and stroke. With regard to the menopause, smokers tend to go through the menopause on average two years earlier than non-smokers and even regular exposure to second-hand smoke can lead to a slightly earlier menopause. Smoking is also associated with an increased risk of developing osteoporosis and increases the likelihood of you having hot flushes, or more severe hot flushes.

The evidence is clear, smoking is not good for you in innumerable ways, but that doesn't mean that it is an easy thing to stop, smoking is an addiction and stopping is hard! There is lots of support available to help you stop smoking including nicotine replacement therapy (which is available on prescription) and support groups. The NHS stop smoking website has lots of information about locally available stop smoking services.

What about e-cigarettes? While I wouldn't recommend that people take up vaping as a healthy habit, it is a valuable tool to help people stop smoking. The health risks associated with e-cigarettes are lower than those associated with smoking cigarettes and switching to vaping is often an effective way of stopping smoking – it means you are still getting the nicotine which is causing the cravings, so you may find that switching is easier in the first instance, and then when you are ready you can gradually reduce these and hopefully stop!

## CHAPTER 5:

# SNEEZING SAFELY! THE PELVIC FLOOR AND URINARY SYSTEM

———◆———

The bladder, urinary system and pelvic floor are all affected by the menopause, with up to 70% of women experiencing some level of symptoms.

There are oestrogen receptors all over the body including in the urinary system, the bladder, the urethra (the tube which urine travels through on its way out of the bladder and into the toilet) and the pelvic floor muscles. The oestrogen-deficient state after the menopause can affect all of these structures as well as the vulva and vagina. The urinary and genital symptoms of the menopause do not usually come on straight away, or during the perimenopause, in the way other symptoms such as hot flushes do (covered in Chapter 4). Instead, these tend to develop more slowly; they are sometimes called "intermediate" symptoms and are related to an ongoing state of low oestrogen.

The genitourinary syndrome of the menopause (GSM) is a term used to encompass both the urinary and genital symptoms related to the menopause and is thought to affect approximately half of postmenopausal women. Genital symptoms such as dryness are covered separately in Chapter 7.

# The pelvic floor

Before we get into the symptoms and changes that happen in the urinary system during the menopause and how to manage them, I want to introduce you to one very important part of the human body: the pelvic floor. We've all heard of it, and we all know we are supposed to exercise it, but most of us absolutely do not, or aren't even sure what it is and what to do next. So let me entice you into this section – doing your pelvic floor exercises helps improve your orgasms! Now I have your attention! And I am doing mine as I write.

The pelvic floor is made up of layers of muscles that cover the bottom of the pelvis, rather like a trampoline, supporting the organs within the pelvis – the bladder, bowel and womb. Ideally, these muscles are firm, thick and strong, like a trampoline as opposed to a hammock. As you move the pelvic floor moves up and down, as do the organs they support. There are three small holes in the trampoline, to allow the urethra (the tube carrying urine from your bladder), the anus and the vagina to pass through. Each of these holes or gaps is generally supported by the pelvic floor muscles holding them tight, like a sphincter. We also have two sphincters at the anus and urethra to give us conscious control of them when we go to the toilet.

## What does the pelvic floor do?

The pelvic floor is a muscle and therefore like any other muscle can be contracted. As you contract the pelvic floor all the organs of the pelvis are lifted up and the sphincters tighten to stop any leakage; relaxing the pelvic floor allows you to go to the toilet. During pregnancy, the pelvic floor provides support for the growing baby and uterus and is involved in labour. Added to this, the pelvic floor, in combination with the back and tummy muscles, works to support and stabilize the spine. Importantly, the pelvic floor muscles are also used for sex, in both men and women, but in women it is the contractions of the pelvic floor which are involved in arousal, sensation and then are part of orgasm.

## Why does the pelvic floor get loose?

The tone of the pelvic floor worsens and the muscles get loose for lots of reasons including pregnancy and childbirth (especially a physically traumatic delivery where there is severe tearing, in particular if the tearing affects the anus), chronic constipation and therefore straining on the toilet, chronic coughing, heavy lifting and even high-impact exercise. Increasing age is unfortunately also a cause, as is having obesity or being overweight. And this section wouldn't be in this book unless the menopause was also involved! As the oestrogen levels fall the pelvic floor weakens, becoming less elastic. As the menopause is often also associated with gaining weight, this can contribute to weakening of the muscle.

*"My kids wrecked my body, I got piles, varicose veins and now I have a pelvic floor like a saggy hammock and can't run for the bus without leaking! Thankfully I love them!"*

Maya, 58

*"I thought I didn't have to do pelvic floor exercises as I haven't been pregnant. Turns out I was wrong!"*

Coleen, 57

## Pelvic floor exercises

*"We are always told to do our pelvic floors, or Kegels, and they say, do them anywhere, the train, at work, at the cinema, but how do you actually do them?"*

Laura, 54

The pelvic floor is made of muscle and we have voluntary control over it, which means, just like with the chest and arms when doing push-ups, we can train and strengthen it. But don't worry, no push-ups are actually involved.

*"Where the hell are they? I am always being told to do my pelvic floors and squeeze, squeeze what?"*

Alice, 47

First of all, you need to find out where the muscles are and how to train them:

◆ Sit or lie down and do the same motion that you would do to stop yourself urinating. If you need to you can try this first when you are actually doing a wee, but this is only to learn the correct sensation, don't keep stopping and starting your urine flow. These are the muscles at the front.

◆ Then do the movement you would do if you were trying to stop passing gas. Imagine you are in an important meeting with your boss and farting would really not be helpful! Squeeze and then relax but don't clench your buttocks at the same time. These are the muscles at the back.

◆ What we are aiming for is a squeezing and lifting sensation. Once you work out where the pelvic floor muscles are, squeeze the front and back together, sort of as if you are trying to hold a tampon in your vagina. Visualizing the area may be useful. Again, don't squeeze your buttocks, tummy or thighs at the same time.

*"Finally an exercise which I can actually do and doesn't involve getting hot and sweaty, jumping around a room with a load of other people!"*

Clare, 51

Now to the exercises themselves. You can do them in any position, lying down, sitting or standing. You may wish to start lying or sitting down and then progress to standing upright. The "floor" of the pelvic floor refers to the position of the muscles at the floor, or bottom of the pelvis – it doesn't mean you have to be sitting or lying on the floor!

◆ **Slow pull-ups.** Squeeze and lift as hard and high as you can, hold and count slowly. Start with a count of 4 or 5 before relaxing but aim to hold the contraction for a slow count of 10. You will need to keep squeezing and contracting actively. Try to tighten a little more with each number you count, as otherwise it is easy to half relax as you count. As you relax you should be aware of a definite lowering or letting go sensation.

- **Fast pull-ups.** We want a strong, stable pelvic floor but we also need it to be able to cope with quick blasts of increased pressure from above, for example during coughing or sneezing. So do quick pull-ups as well, holding for a count of one or two before relaxing.

- Keep breathing, keep counting and keep focusing on not using your buttocks or thighs.

- Aim for ten repetitions of each exercise.

Most patient information leaflets will say to aim for three times a day and that pelvic floor exercises are hidden so you can do them anywhere. Of course this is true, but let's be realistic, start by putting a Post-it note on your bathroom mirror or lid of your moisturizer with a reminder. In the beginning aim for twice a day. Putting that reminder on something that you automatically use twice a day, like on your toothpaste when brushing your teeth, can be useful. After all, two full sets of effective exercises will be more effective than three half-hearted 2-minute attempts while trying to concentrate on something else! The whole set should take about 5 minutes and in time you can increase how often you do them.

Once you have mastered a slow and quick pull-up you can make the exercises harder. Don't stop doing the slow and quick pulls but you can add in the following two exercises:

- Imagine that your vagina is a lift and the relaxed position is the ground floor. Now pull up one third to the first floor and pause, then the next third to the second floor and pause, and then all the way up to the top. Squeeze at the top then relax all the way down.

◆ And then the hardest one: lift all the way to the top and imagine the lift is going back down again, one floor (or one third) at a time, keeping control all the way.

Both these exercises can also be repeated ten times each, with every set of pelvic floor exercises you do.

Pelvic floor exercises do work, but they are not always easy to do. Up to about half of women struggle with the technique, so if you don't notice an improvement then please visit your GP who will be able to refer you to a women's health physiotherapist.

It doesn't matter how old you are, whether or not you have been doing them your whole life, or never; just start and then keep going. We can never stop!

## The bladder and incontinence

As you age, and therefore the further you are from when you went through the menopause, the bladder becomes smaller and less elastic. This means that you need to go to the toilet more frequently and it can even lead to urge incontinence (see page 132). Add in weakening of the pelvic floor and stress incontinence (see page 128) can occur. The urethra also becomes thin, meaning it is even easier for bacteria to get into your bladder, resulting in urine infections. Urine infections are more common in women than men, due to the short urethra and small distance between the anus and urethra in comparison to men. After the menopause the natural acidity of the vagina changes, allowing more bacteria to flourish, again increasing the risk of urinary tract infections. Urinary symptoms are also more common in women who smoke, so stopping smoking can be useful for both urinary symptoms as well as your general health.

*"I get it, I am supposed to exercise. But I can't. I will just wet myself. I can't."*

Sophia, 56

*"I am 58 and wearing a pad in case of leaks, this alone makes me feel 100."*

Cassie, 58

Let me say this. Incontinence is not a "natural" part of ageing, it is not something you have to live with, you do not have to accept wearing a pad in case of leaks as part of your life. Go and speak to your doctor. There are treatments that can help. And I get it, the thought of going to talk about wetting yourself is mortifying, but we must keep talking about it, so that women can get the help they need and deserve. If you do use a pad, perhaps while waiting for your pelvic floor exercises to work, use a pad designed to hold urine as sanitary towels cannot hold enough volume.

Your bladder is a balloon made of muscle. The kidneys produce urine as a constant slow trickle which is carried through two tubes called the ureters to the bladder. But we don't go to the toilet as a slow constant trickle; instead the bladder slowly expands as it fills with urine. Another tube, the urethra, is the outlet pipe, but there is a sphincter at the top of the urethra – a tight band of muscle which is held closed until you go to the toilet and voluntarily decide to open it, allowing you to urinate. That sphincter is supported by the pelvic floor muscles. When the bladder is holding around 300–400 ml of urine, messages are sent to the brain that you need to go. As you go to the toilet, the sphincter opens, the bladder contracts and the pelvic floor muscles relax, and voila, the joy of peeing, when you really need to go!

Incontinence is when you release urine without meaning to, and it is really common – about one in five women over the age of 40 will be affected, but in reality this number is likely to be higher as many women do not discuss it. There are various types of incontinence. The two commonest are stress incontinence and urge incontinence, though you can have a mixed pattern combining both. See your doctor to rule out an infection and so you can get treatment.

## Stress incontinence

Have you ever run after a bus and had to stop because you were worried you were going to leak? Or worried about doing an exercise class involving jumping because you will wet yourself? How confident are you coughing or sneezing, that you won't wet yourself at the same time? Or even have you just found yourself constantly running to the toilet?

*"I don't think that I will totally wet myself, with floods dripping down my legs, but a slight dribble is just as worrying. If I have a cough or a cold I just can't trust that I won't dribble and then I really worry about a smell. I have started wearing a pad all the time, and I hate it."*

Helena, 54

*"You know the saying about laughing so much that you wet yourself? That happens to me every time I laugh at all!"*

Iris, 58

Urinary incontinence means the involuntary leaking of urine, be it a little or a lot, and tends to occur during:

◆ Coughing.

◆ Sneezing.

◆ Laughing.

◆ Exercise – running/jumping, anything involving impact generally.

## Why?

Stress incontinence is the commonest form of incontinence and occurs when you leak urine as the pressure in or on the bladder is increased. If the support of the pelvic floor is weakened, such as after the menopause, stress incontinence becomes more likely.

## What can I do?

For many women, the combination of the following can be enough to control symptoms:

◆ The mainstay of treatment for stress incontinence is pelvic floor exercises.

◆ Stop smoking.

◆ Lose weight.

If pelvic floor exercises aren't working or aren't enough then see your doctor; they will be able to refer you to a women's health physiotherapist, who will be able to help you with the exercises and may also use the following:

◆ Biofeedback – this helps you exercise the correct muscles. A small device is inserted into the vagina. When you exercise correctly a noise is made, or a light flashes on the computer, giving you feedback that you are doing the pelvic floor exercises correctly (as they are hard!).

◆ Vaginal weights or cones – small weighted plastic cones that you put in your vagina and then hold in for 10–15 mins. Generally the exercise is done two to three times a day. You start with a very light cone and work your way up. This is not the same as using the infamous vaginal jade eggs; there are no known health benefits from using jade eggs!

◆ Electrical stimulation – a small device is inserted into the vagina, which stimulates the pelvic floor to contract, helping it to get stronger.

*"I am a weightlifter you know! I lift weights, with my vagina!"*

Renee, 56

## Medication

A medication called duloxetine may be offered if pelvic floor exercises alone are not enough to control any symptoms. It is an antidepressant medicine but appears to help stress incontinence whether or not you are depressed, by stimulating the nerve controlling the sphincter at the top of the urethra, keeping it closed. It doesn't cure incontinence, but about 60% of women reported that they leaked about half the number of times when taking duloxetine compared to when they weren't taking the medication.

Topical vaginal oestrogen may also be helpful. For more information please see page 172.

## Surgery

Surgery is generally only offered when pelvic floor exercises have not helped. By supporting the muscles below the bladder it is possible to treat stress incontinence.

◆ A common surgery recently used is tension free vaginal tape (TVT), where a small sling is inserted to support the neck of the bladder. The number of these surgeries is likely to fall as there has recently been evidence that surgery using tapes or meshes can cause severe long-term complications such as chronic pelvic pain, bladder or bowel symptoms such as incontinence or pain, vaginal bleeding and problems with sexual intercourse. As such, non-surgical options are generally considered first. If surgery is performed, using mesh is generally not the first choice, but if it is being offered then you should be given information about the potential risks of the surgery and should be followed up by the surgeon.

◆ Colposuspension – here the tissues around the bladder are lifted up to help support it.

◆ If you have a prolapse, surgery to repair this can also be effective in treating stress incontinence.

◆ Injections into the urethral sphincter are used to try to keep it closed, using silicone or fat.

# Overactive bladder and urge incontinence

Not all incontinence is "stress incontinence", indeed there may be leakage of urine without coughing or sneezing.

*"My doctor said I had latchkey urgency, basically I needed to go all the time, but had an unbearable need the moment I put the key in the door. I had to dump my bag and coat and run before saying hello to anyone."*

Cara, 59

Symptoms of overactive bladder can include:

◆ Frequency – going to the toilet far more than usual, generally more than eight times a day.

◆ Nocturia – waking up more than once a night to go to the toilet.

◆ Urgency – a sudden, urgent need to go to the toilet, you can't wait, you need to go now!

◆ Urge incontinence – this doesn't always occur with an overactive bladder but can do, where you leak urine before getting to the toilet in time. The volume of urine can be anything from a little to a lot.

## Why?

Overactive bladder syndrome, or detrusor instability, is a condition in which the bladder suddenly contracts, whether or not the bladder is full. You have no control over the contractions. The cause of an overactive bladder is not always known, but it often appears after the menopause as the bladder becomes smaller and less elastic or stretchy. It can also occur due to a brain or nerve problem such as a stroke or MS.

## What can I do?

*"I thought the less I drank the better it would be, the less I drank the less urine I would make surely, but actually it made it worse. I went just as often, if not more often, but only a tiny amount came out each time."*

Elaine, 61

- Start with simple things – make it as easy as possible to get to the toilet quickly, especially at night, without tripping over rugs and chairs and other things in the way!
- Keep up your fluid intake – it often feels like cutting down on the amount of fluid you drink would help, but this isn't the case. Firstly, the bladder contracts in overactive bladder syndrome even when it isn't full. Secondly, the less you drink the more concentrated the urine becomes, so even if it is a small amount it can irritate the bladder, worsening the spasms or contractions. So keep drinking as normal.
- Weight loss – even losing a small amount of weight can help with symptoms as there is less pressure on the bladder.
- Cut down on caffeine and alcohol. Caffeine is a diuretic; it makes you produce more urine. It can also stimulate the bladder muscle, so the combination of more urine and an additional stimulation to the bladder can worsen symptoms. Try going caffeine free! Alcohol is also a diuretic and can worsen your symptoms. If you don't want to go alcohol or caffeine free, at least be aware that symptoms may worsen when ingesting these substances and plan to be near a toilet.

◆ Only go to the toilet when you need to – going more often to try to prevent the urgency means that the bladder gets less and less used to being stretched and holding more urine. This means that when it is stretched a little bit, the urgency becomes worse.

◆ Bladder training (bladder drill) – the mainstay of treatment, which aims to stretch the bladder slowly so it can hold more urine so you need to go less often. You will be advised on bladder training by a healthcare professional.

- Initially you keep a diary of when and how much urine you pass for a couple of days.
- You will be encouraged to hold on and delay passing urine when you need to, initially by a small amount of time such as 5 minutes, which is then gradually increased.
- Over a few weeks you should be able to hold on for longer periods of time and eventually go only five to six times a day passing larger amounts of urine.

◆ Medication:

- Antimuscarinic medication such as oxybutynin, solifenacin or tolterodine may be prescribed. They work to relax the bladder to stop contractions.
- The combination of medication and bladder training is often very effective.
- Again, topical vaginal oestrogen may be helpful. See page 172 for more.
- Botox – not just for wrinkles! Injections of botulinum toxin into the bladder can help to relax the muscle if other medications and bladder training have not been effective.

Nerve stimulation – various nerves can be stimulated to try to control the muscle of the bladder again, if other treatments have been ineffective. It involves a small probe or device inserted into the vagina or anus to stimulate the nerves of the lower back and pelvic floor.

## Mixed incontinence

For many people the picture is mixed, a combination of stress and urgency incontinence. If it isn't clear your doctor may refer you for urodynamic tests. These involve measuring the pressure in the bladder as it fills after you drink a large amount of water. It then measures how much urine is passed when you go and if anything is left in the bladder. Often a combination of treatments is needed.

# Urinary tract infections (UTIs)

*"We all know it, right? The burning when you pee, like peeing through glass or razor blades, and then the need to go all the time, and I mean all the time. Yet another UTI."*

Natalie, 53

Symptoms of a urinary tract infection can include:

◆ Frequency and nocturia – needing to go to the toilet more often than usual, and/or at night.
◆ Urgency – an urgent need to go!
◆ Dysuria – pain, stinging or burning on passing urine.
◆ Pain or pressure in the pelvis or lower back.
◆ Cloudy or smelly urine.
◆ Blood in the urine.

- Feeling tired.
- Shivering or shaking with fever – this may indicate that the infection has spread to the kidneys.

## Why?

Urine infections are common, especially in women, where the urethra is short, allowing easy passage of bacteria from around the anus into the bladder. This is exacerbated by the thinning of the urethra after the menopause. Add to this the change in vaginal acidity after the menopause, allowing more bacteria to grow in the vagina and thinning of all the genital tissue, and urine infections are common.

## What can I do?

Your doctor will test your urine for blood, protein, white blood cells and nitrites (nitrites are formed from a naturally occurring substance in the urine called nitrates, by the presence of bacteria). Your doctor may also send the sample of urine to the lab to try to grow the bacteria and then see which antibiotic the bacteria is sensitive to. Your GP will generally treat a urine infection with a short course of antibiotics.

- Drink plenty of fluids.
- Don't douche or wash inside the vagina, as it can encourage bacteria up around and into the urethra and bladder. It also isn't good for your vagina, as it washes away any good bacteria! Similarly, perfumed soaps, bubble baths and talcum powders should be avoided as they can irritate the skin.

◆ Ensure that you have enough lubrication during sex as dryness increases the friction, which then leads to inflammation, increasing the risk of infection. For more information on lubrication during sex please see page 169.

If you have recurrent infections the following may be offered:

◆ A blood test for diabetes, as UTIs are more common if there is sugar in the urine, as in diabetes. Controlling the diabetes can help prevent the infections.

◆ Topical oestrogen – using oestrogen creams or gel pessaries in the vagina can be extremely useful in preventing UTIs. They work by improving the quality of the tissues of the vagina, vulva and urethra and change the pH of the vagina back to the pre-menopausal state and so help prevent urine infections. For more information about topical oestrogen please see page 172.

◆ Sometimes longer courses of antibiotics are also needed.

*"To be honest I didn't believe my GP when she said that oestrogen cream in my vagina could help stop the urine infections, but as the months went by without an infection I started to change my mind. And to be honest, sex is better too!"*

Fran, 56

# Prolapse

A prolapse is when one organ in the pelvis (or sometimes more) bulges into the vagina.

◆ A mild prolapse may have no symptoms.

- A womb prolapse may lead to a dragging, aching sensation in the vagina, or pelvic pain. If severe, there may be a bulge of tissue hanging out of the vagina.
- The bladder or bowel can be affected, worsening or leading to urinary urgency or incontinence, or a feeling that you haven't completely emptied your bladder, or bowel problems such as constipation or a feeling you haven't completely opened your bowels. Some women insert a finger or a Femmeze device into the vagina in order to push the prolapse back in order to empty the bladder or bowel fully.
- Frequent urine infections.
- Painful sex.

*"I had visions of my grandmother when the doctor said I had a prolapse, and they weren't good. I knew she often literally pushed her womb back in again! Thankfully the doctor said there were things we could do."*

Eva, 64

## Why?

Your pelvic floor muscles work to hold up the organs in your pelvis, which are also supported by various strong ligaments. If the pelvic floor and these ligaments become weak, for example after the menopause, the organs sag downwards with gravity, generally into the vagina, resulting in a prolapse. Other risk factors include pregnancy, childbirth and obesity.

There are various types of prolapse depending on the organ which is sagging down – the uterus, bowel, bladder or urethra can be affected.

## What can I do?

*"Doing my pelvic floor exercises really helped, now I do them religiously."*

Ellie, 54

- Weight loss can help prolapse symptoms, by decreasing the amount of pressure on the pelvic floor from the abdomen.
- Constipation makes symptoms worse, so trying to avoid this can be helpful. Try eating 1–2 tablespoons of linseeds per day, sprinkled on yoghurt or cereal as the fibre involved is often enough to help you go regularly. If not, see your pharmacist or GP for advice on laxatives.
- Pelvic floor exercises – these can really help the symptoms, please see page 123.
- Surgery – there are various operations available depending on the type and severity of the prolapse.
- Pessaries – a plastic pessary can be inserted into the vagina to help support the pelvic floor. These are generally only used in older women if surgery isn't appropriate.

*"No one wants an operation but I had tried it all, I did my pelvic floor exercises religiously and took the medicines but they weren't enough and it was really affecting me. Having surgery was the right choice for me, all my symptoms have gone!"*

Naeve, 56

## SUMMARY POINTS

- The pelvic floor is a hammock of muscles holding up the organs in the pelvis.
- Doing pelvic floor exercises daily can improve the strength of the pelvic floor and improve urinary symptoms.
- Stress incontinence is when there is urine leakage on coughing/straining/laughing/jumping, anything where there is an increase in abdominal pressure. It is generally treated with pelvic floor strengthening, though surgery may be required.
- Urge incontinence or detrusor overactivity is where the bladder contracts whether or not it is full. It is generally treated with bladder training and medication.
- The two types of incontinence can occur together.
- Prolapse is when one or more of the organs of the pelvic floor sags into the vagina. It is generally treated with pelvic floor strengthening, and sometimes surgical treatment.

# CHAPTER 6:

# MENSTRUAL MAYHEM

———◆———

Many women are surprised by the change in their bleeding in the perimenopause, somehow expecting that the periods would just drift further and further apart, becoming lighter and lighter before stopping. While that is the case for some women, for others their periods go out in a blaze of glory, getting – sometimes dramatically – heavier and more frequent!

*"My periods came like clockwork, 29 days apart at 11 a.m., literally within a few minutes of when I expected, to the extent that I would just pop in a pad at 10.30 a.m. and know I was sorted. So I find the irregularity really difficult, always carrying tampons or pads, often wearing a panty liner, just in case."*

Carrie, 48

## Changes in bleeding pattern

So there you are, in your 20s and 30s with your period coming more or less when you expect it, but in your 40s, things may well begin to change, and there is no predicting exactly what that change may be.

Having no change at all, or a slight change to the cycle length, with it often becoming slightly shorter at 25 or 26 days, but sometimes longer by a few days, is common. But with regular periods, even if they come ever so slightly more often, your ovaries are still working regularly.

For some women the periods will get lighter and less frequent gradually over time. This in itself can be confusing and difficult, as you don't know when they are coming yet there is also the possibility of pregnancy – so if you are not using an extremely reliable source of contraception such as the coil, you will still need to consider that a lack of a period may well mean a pregnancy and not the menopause (see Chapter 8 for more on safe sex during the menopause).

For others, the periods continue regularly until one day they just stop. But as the menopause is a diagnosis of retrospect, we still won't be able to know for sure that you have been through the menopause until you have not bled for one year.

And for others the periods come more and more frequently, getting closer and closer together. They may last longer and/or get heavier, which can cause distress and embarrassment, with flooding and passing clots. The heavier periods can also be more painful than before.

*"It was like the flood gates had opened, one minute I was sitting in a meeting and the next I stood up and realized I had totally soaked through my trousers all over the chair. I don't think anyone noticed before I did, I just sat down again and waited for everyone to leave, praying that they wouldn't see."*

Emily, 49

The older you get the fewer follicles there are in the ovaries, and the follicles that you do have left become less and less responsive to follicle-stimulating hormone (FSH), which is why FSH levels rise as the brain tries to pump more FSH to stimulate the ovaries. The less responsive a follicle is, the longer it may take to mature, so the gap between periods can become longer and longer. (See page 23 for further explanation of the menstrual cycle.)

Sometimes you will get an "anovulatory" cycle, which means a cycle without ovulation, so the ovaries are functioning but not functioning properly. (This can happen at any time during your life, but is more likely during puberty and climacteria.) In this situation, the follicles have responded to FSH but not produced an egg, but they still produce oestrogen, leading the lining of the womb to build up. As no egg has been produced there is no corpus luteum (the shell of the follicle from which the egg popped out), which means that no progesterone is produced. Oestrogen and progesterone ordinarily work together to build up and maintain the lining of the womb; when the progesterone levels fall, your period starts. But in an anovulatory cycle there is no progesterone, so the oestrogen keeps stimulating the lining of the womb to build up and up and up. This thick lining eventually becomes unstable and breaks down, but as it was so thick the period can be hugely heavy and long, with women describing periods of up to ten days or more. There may be flooding through protection, or you may feel you need to wear multiple products such as a tampon/cup and a sanitary towel/period pants to protect against this. You may also need to change much more frequently than previously and may pass clots.

# How heavy is too heavy?

We can't blame everything on the perimenopause, both with regard to irregular and heavy periods. Anovulatory cycles are irregular, so if you are regularly having much heavier periods there may be another cause. Your periods may be irregular due to a thyroid issue or even due to the kind of contraception you are using, and heavy periods may be due to fibroids, which are benign growths in the womb.

*"I was always taught to not make a fuss, just keep going. So I felt embarrassed about going to the doctor to say that my periods had got heavy and painful, what if they said they weren't heavy and I was just being a bit pathetic?"*

Sharon, 52

How heavy your periods are, or how heavy you feel they are, is your judgement call and what is normal for one woman may be heavy for you. No one is going to ask you to collect the blood or weigh your pads to work out if you are bleeding more or less than the next person. Some women were asked to do so for the sake of research, with the results showing that blood loss in an average period is 20–40 ml (4–8 teaspoons) and a heavy period being over 80 ml (16 teaspoons).

Your periods would be considered to be heavy if you are soaking through your sanitary protection despite changing it regularly; need to wear both tampons and pads, or multiple forms of sanitary protection, to prevent flooding your clothes or bed; need to change your pad/tampon/cup every 1–2 hours and/or are passing large clots (larger than about an inch or a 10p coin); or if your periods last longer than a week. Even if they don't meet these criteria but are heavier than normal for you and you feel that you aren't managing, then please see your doctor for help and treatment!

# What happens next?

*"I thought my doctor would say it was the change and that I had to deal with it, but I was worried that something else was going on. She arranged a scan and thankfully there wasn't, but just knowing that there was nothing else made me feel better."*

Charlotte, 46

As mentioned on page 40, the blood test to check FSH levels in the menopause is not generally useful. However, your doctor may request blood tests to check your thyroid function, as low thyroid hormone levels can cause heavy periods. They may also check a full blood count and ferritin levels to investigate anaemia and iron storage respectively, in the body.

Your doctor may examine you by feeling your tummy but also by performing an internal vaginal examination. With one hand on top of the tummy and two fingers in the vagina your doctor can feel your womb between their two hands. They may also do a speculum examination (just like for a smear test) to check if they can see a polyp, a generally benign growth, in the cervix. They may also request an ultrasound scan of the pelvis to check and see if there are any fibroids, polyps or if the lining of the womb has become too thick. An ultrasound scan is the same scan that pregnant women have, using sound waves (at too high a frequency for you to hear) to visualize organs as the sound waves bounce back off the organs, but for the best view of the organs in the pelvis it is often performed transvaginally, through the vagina. Here a small probe is covered with a sterile condom-type covering and gently inserted into the vagina. This may be uncomfortable but shouldn't be painful; if it is too uncomfortable or you would prefer not to have a transvaginal scan you can have the scan by placing the probe over the tummy.

Depending on the results, if it is thought, for example, that you may have a polyp you may be referred to the hospital to have a hysteroscopy, which is where a small camera is inserted through the cervix to visualize the womb. This can be done under local or general anaesthetic.

# What can be done?

*"I was willing to try anything to be honest. Every three weeks I was too frightened to go out as I was changing pads every hour and sitting on a towel in case I leaked. I would set my alarm to wake up three times in the night to change my pads."*

Mel, 50

If your periods are getting more and more irregular and lighter then no treatment for the periods themselves is needed, though of course you may wish to consider treatment for other symptoms. But if the periods are getting longer, heavier and more frequent then there are various treatment options available.

If your heavy bleeding has caused anaemia, it is generally treated by a combination of attending to the cause of the bleeding but also iron replacement. And if you are given iron tablets then they can cause constipation, but don't worry if they make your poo turn black! Also take them with vitamin C or a glass of orange juice as the vitamin C in the juice helps you absorb the iron.

## Tranexamic acid

Tranexamic acid is an antifibrinolytic drug that works by decreasing the amount of bleeding you have, slowing the breakdown of blood clots. It makes your bleeding not only less heavy but also often shorter. It does not involve any hormones at all and tends not to have any significant side effects.

The dose is generally 1 g, which is taken as two 500 mg tablets three times a day. You start taking it on day 1 of your period and can take it for a maximum of four days, so even if you are still bleeding on day 5 you must stop taking it, but if you stop bleeding after three days you don't need to take all four days' worth!

You can take tranexamic acid on its own or in combination with a non-steroidal anti-inflammatory drug, and the combination is often very effective.

## Non-steroidal anti-inflammatory drugs (NSAIDs)

NSAIDs include medications such as ibuprofen and naproxen, though the one most commonly prescribed for heavy and/or painful periods is mefenamic acid. NSAIDs work by making the body produce less of a substance called prostaglandins which are involved in heavy periods and help to relieve pain. If you get "preperiod pain", pain before the bleeding starts, you can start taking this type of medication straight away, you do not need to wait for the bleeding to start. In fact, starting painkillers earlier, before the pain gets too severe, often means that you need less medication to bring the pain under control.

As mentioned already, you can take mefenamic acid in combination with tranexamic acid and the two together often work effectively.

If you have asthma which is triggered by medications like ibuprofen, or find your asthma is worse after taking mefenamic acid, then please stop taking it. In addition, if you have a gastrointestinal condition, such as an ulcer or even severe indigestion you may be advised not to take the medication as NSAIDs can irritate the stomach.

## Combined oral contraceptive pill

The combined oral contraceptive pill is covered in more detail on page 187. It stops ovulation and is often used as a treatment for heavy periods as the bleed related to the pill is a withdrawal bleed as you withdraw from the hormones in the pill. However, the latest guidance information about the combined pill states that you don't need to have a pill-free break at all and no pill-free break means no period! At some point, you may notice some spotting, and if you have spotting for four days consecutively, have a four-day pill-free break and then restart.

The combined oral contraceptive pill does contain hormones and, as long as there are no other risk factors such as smoking, can be used up until the age of 50. It gets bonus points as it also works as contraception and can help relieve other menopausal symptoms.

## Cyclical progesterone

The heavy periods of an anovulatory cycle are thought to be related to a lack of progesterone, so taking progesterone for the second two weeks of each cycle should help control how often the periods come, though the flow may still be heavy. However, if you have risk factors meaning that you cannot take the combined pill, cyclical progesterone may be suitable and it can be used until the periods stop.

## Intrauterine system – hormone-containing coil

An intrauterine system (IUS) is a progesterone-containing coil (more information available on page 194). There are various types available which last for varying lengths of time but the most commonly used is the Mirena coil. The Mirena IUS also gets bonus points as it has the added advantage of being licensed for use as the progesterone part of HRT (see page 239) should you need and want it and is a form of contraception.

It works by making the lining of the womb very thin and a thinner lining means less bleeding. In fact, after one year's use 90% of women have no bleeding at all. However, in the first few months there can be irregular spotting, which in some women is more continuous, though this can be treated with additional oral progesterone and generally settles down.

*"I didn't believe that it could work. The doctor showed me one before he put it in, how could a little plastic anchor stop the torrents that my periods had become? I wanted a hysterectomy to be honest but the Mirena changed all that, I barely bled for about four months, but since then have had nothing at all, and I don't need to worry about contraception – win win!"*

*Rachel, 47*

## Surgery

If the heavy bleeding does not respond to any of the above and an ultrasound scan was normal (or showed only small fibroids) you may be referred to a gynaecologist to consider an endometrial ablation or resection. This is generally performed as a day case under general anaesthetic. The procedure destroys the lining of the womb and without a lining there will be less bleeding and often none at all, though in a minority of cases it isn't effective.

If none of the above methods have worked, or if you have large fibroids and so an endometrial ablation is not appropriate, sometimes a hysterectomy is offered. Women with large fibroids who are still trying to conceive are sometimes offered a different operation, a myomectomy where just the fibroids are removed. However, this is more likely to cause bleeding during the operation so if you are older or are sure you are not planning to become pregnant then a hysterectomy may be offered instead. Depending on the size of any fibroids a hysterectomy can be performed vaginally (if the fibroids are very small) or through the abdomen, often as a keyhole surgery. This is a major surgery so is generally only considered if other options have not worked, and the number being performed has fallen since treatments such as the Mirena coil have become available.

# HRT and periods

If you start HRT when you are still having periods – which you can do to control your symptoms – you will be offered a sequential form of HRT (see page 238). This means that you are given oestrogen daily and progesterone for the last two weeks of every cycle and most people will then have a period each month, generally at the beginning of next month's pack. An alternative is to use the Mirena coil to control the bleeding and then oestrogen to control the menopausal symptoms.

If the periods have stopped before you start HRT you will be put on a continuous combined regimen. This may cause some spotting for the first four to six months but should then not cause bleeding at all.

If you were started on sequential HRT at some point you will be switched to a continuous combined form, sometimes after a year or two of being on HRT, or after the age of 55. Your doctor will discuss with you at your HRT review the best time to switch to continuous combined, as depending on your circumstances the change can be earlier, if you have been taking the sequential form for at least a year and are thought to not have any functioning ovarian tissue left.

## Bleeding after sex and in between periods

The first part of this chapter was about the fact that your bleeding may go a bit all over the place in the perimenopause, coming further and further apart or closer and closer together or just irregular. But don't assume that all changes are related to the perimenopause: if you have bleeding in between your periods or after sex you should go and see your doctor as this could signify another issue such as an infection or a polyp, or it can be a symptom of something more serious such as cancer.

# Postmenopausal bleeding

Postmenopausal bleeding (PMB) is defined as bleeding from the vagina which occurs after the menopause, so 12 months after you have had no bleeding at all.

There are various possible causes of postmenopausal bleeding including womb (endometrial), cervical, vulval, vaginal or ovarian cancer. Other causes include polyps in the womb or cervix, as well as non-cancerous thickening of the lining of the womb (called endometrial hyperplasia). Thinning of the skin of the vagina, known as vaginal atrophy, can also lead to postmenopausal bleeding, though often in smaller amounts (further information on vaginal atrophy, also called atrophic vaginitis, can be found in Chapter 9). HRT can also cause vaginal bleeding as described above.

## What should I do?

If you notice postmenopausal bleeding then please arrange an urgent appointment with your GP. Unless an obvious cause is found, for example after an injury or trauma, you are likely to be referred on a two-week wait referral to see a gynaecologist in a local hospital. A two-week wait referral is a "suspected cancer" referral, but this doesn't mean that you have cancer; rather, you have a symptom that could indicate cancer, though in the majority of cases it will not be. At the hospital you will see a gynaecologist who will take a history and examine you and you are likely to have an ultrasound scan. After the menopause, the lining of the womb is thin, much thinner than before the menopause, so if it becomes thicker again it will need to be investigated. The doctor may take a sample of the lining of the womb through your cervix using a tiny pipette, sometimes while you are awake in the outpatient department. A hysteroscopy may also be performed, under local or general anaesthetic, where a tiny camera is inserted through the cervix into the womb to look for polyps or other lesions which can then be removed.

If endometrial cancer is found, then depending on the extent, often a hysterectomy is offered, with the tubes and ovaries being removed at the same time. Radiotherapy and chemotherapy may also be offered.

*"To be honest I was more surprised than scared when I started bleeding again and nearly didn't go to the doctor but something niggled that I should. I mean I hadn't seen my period for about three years. I had a scan and they found a polyp which they then removed. All done!"*

Ruth, 55

## SUMMARY POINTS

- For some women, their periods will become lighter and more irregular, getting further and further apart before stopping.
- For others, their periods will get much heavier and come more frequently.

- Treatments for heavy periods include medication such as tranexamic acid, the contraceptive pill or a hormone-delivering coil (IUS/Mirena device). Surgical options are also available.
- If you start HRT while you are still having periods you will be given a form of HRT known as sequential HRT, which still gives withdrawal bleeds.
- If your periods have stopped when you start HRT, you will be given continuous combined HRT, which does not lead to withdrawal bleeds.
- Postmenopausal bleeding – bleeding after no periods for one year must always be investigated by your doctor.

## CHAPTER 7:

# LET'S TALK ABOUT SEX (AND RELATIONSHIPS)

———◆———

Let's talk about sex. Except actually, we don't! Sex is still a taboo, especially women enjoying sex, or desiring sex, but even more so, not enjoying it and not wanting it. And postmenopausal sex is probably an even greater taboo. Be honest, would you talk to your friends about vaginal dryness during sex, or about the best lubricant to use? Most people don't, but actually this is a huge topic, which affects so many women during the perimenopause and beyond and we need to talk about it more. If we were more comfortable talking about sex, desire and pleasure, perhaps we would be more comfortable asking for help when things aren't going to plan.

Young people don't tend to think of older people as having sex lives, yet data from the English Longitudinal Study of Ageing showed that over half of men (54%) and about a third of women (31%) are sexually active over the age of 70, with about a third of these men and women having regular sex; and a US-based study showed 70% of couples over the age of 75 have sex at least once per week. For many people, sex matters. It is an important part of a relationship in many ways, not simply for sexual gratification but for intimacy and closeness. Regular sex has other benefits: it boosts mood, can help sleep and relaxation, and reduces the risk of depression. It is a physical activity, a form of exercise, and has physical health benefits, too, boosting your immune system. Not forgetting the fact that it feels good and makes you feel good!

I ask any woman with perimenopausal or menopausal symptoms who comes to see me about sex, about their sex drive and whether or not sex is painful. I preface it by saying that I ask everyone these questions because they can be difficult to bring up. For many of my patients, it is the first time anyone has asked them these questions and they often say that they feel relieved to have been given permission to talk about it. For others though, it is a surprise as they seem to assume that it is part and parcel of growing older, that their libidos should fall. But it doesn't have to be! There are lots of things that we can do to help so please, please come forward and ask for the help you need, and then, ladies, spread the word. You can have sex, you can want to have sex and you can enjoy sex without discomfort, no matter your age. After all, the menopause isn't an ending, it is a beginning, a new start to a new phase in your life, with as much (safe!) sex as you want.

# Libido

*"But I don't want it. To be honest I am happier with a box set and a pizza!"*

Lynda, 50

Libido, or sex drive, is a complicated thing, involving many physical and psychological factors. Think about it – if you don't feel well with a cold or something, you aren't keen on sex; or if you are feeling sad or anxious, you don't feel like sex; or if things aren't great in your relationship, you don't want to have sex; or last time it hurt, so why would you want to have sex? Or you're tired, or hungry, or annoyed, or, or, or. In fact, when I ask my patients about sex they often respond with something like "What sex?"

*"My sex drive seemed to vanish somewhere into the ether, I don't know exactly when or why, but it has gone. It all just seems like a bother now."*

Mel, 49

## What can I do?

Loss of libido, or sexual desire, is thought to affect about half of women during the perimenopause and menopause and it isn't really surprising. Before we even consider the effects of the change in hormones on your desire itself we have to consider all the other factors – the fatigue and exhaustion, irritability, mood swings, feeling low or anxious, joints aching, sweats and more. Add into the mix vaginal dryness, leading to painful sex (more on page 166) and your libido can disappear.

*"It is really beginning to affect my relationship. I loved sex before, I mean I really did and we had a great sex life, but now I can take it or leave it, he feels that me not initiating any more is a rejection."*

Paula, 48

*"I lost all my impetus to have any kind of sexual contact at all. My girlfriend is a bit older than me but her libido wasn't affected during the menopause so she didn't really understand why mine was. To be honest it is causing an issue between us."*

Tanya, 48

Many people will have sex when they aren't really in the mood for it, perhaps because sometimes they need to start in order to feel desire, perhaps to please a partner, or because they enjoy other feelings that it gives apart from sexual pleasure. However, aside from the issue of libido or desire, after the menopause many women report that even when they do have sex, it simply doesn't feel as good as it did before, that arousal is not as easy or takes longer, that it is less satisfying, or it is more difficult to reach orgasm. For some women, this is due to vaginal dryness (see page 165) or painful sex but it can occur alone.

*"It's normal though, right? I mean you go at it like rabbits, then along come the babies and you are just too knackered to do anything, and then eventually they grow up a bit and you can put a lock on the bedroom door and you get back into it. It's all tailed off a bit again, but I thought that was to be expected. Boy was my partner happy when things changed!"*

Sal, 51

## Why?

You know the answer by now – hormones! But not just falling levels of oestrogen; when it comes to libido, testosterone is also involved. You may think of testosterone as being the "male" hormone, but actually women produce it too, though in smaller amounts. About half of your testosterone is made in the ovaries, but even if the ovaries are not removed surgically, perhaps due to cancer, levels fall, which may be due to a change in the blood supply to the ovaries. Testosterone is also made in the adrenal glands, which are found just on top of each kidney. Testosterone is produced in the ovaries from puberty, but the amount produced gradually falls, so by the time you reach the menopause your levels are about half of what they were at the peak in your 20s. So levels are already falling, irrespective of the menopause. You still produce testosterone after the menopause, and without the high levels of oestrogen the testosterone can dominate, for example producing hair growth on your face or hair loss on your scalp. But this "unmasking" of the testosterone doesn't seem to influence libido; it doesn't give the boost to your sex drive that you otherwise might expect. In fact, the low levels of testosterone, even if you factor in the low levels of oestrogen, seem to trigger a fall in your libido.

Testosterone has other functions apart from in sex drive. It is also involved in arousal and the sexual response to stimulation by increasing levels of a chemical in the nervous system named dopamine, which is a feel-good chemical. Aside from sex, it seems to be involved in metabolism, bone and muscle strength, fatigue and energy levels, heart health, memory and concentration and just feeling good! Low testosterone levels can also lead to headaches.

## What can I do?

As sex drive is such a complicated matter, increasing your libido isn't always as simple as taking a little blue pill and going to bed! In fact, a female Viagra could be considered a pharmaceutical company's holy grail, as it could potentially make a killing!

But there are things that can help.

Firstly, it is important to consider any physical issues that could be affecting your sex drive, and for menopausal women this is often vaginal dryness and/or pain during sex. And this one we can fix, often pretty easily (for more information please see page 169–175).

Your doctor can also look at any medication you may be on, as some medications can affect libido. Mental health problems such as depression also affect sex drive, so treating this can have a positive effect, but low testosterone may also cause depression, so it is complicated.

A blood test is not required for diagnosis of decreased libido (hypoactive sexual desire disorder), but it can be useful to show low testosterone levels. Doctors may use a blood test to monitor response to testosterone replacement, perhaps requesting an initial blood test and then a repeat test three to six months later.

## Testosterone replacement

If low testosterone is part of the problem then it seems sensible to assume that replacing the testosterone would solve the problem. And for some women it can really help, not just with libido and sexual arousal, but with boosting energy, concentration, focus and stamina. There may be improvements in your muscle mass, strength and memory, as well as an improvement in mood. You might notice the sensation of feeling back to your normal self, or a general sense of well-being. A study published in *The Lancet* in July

2019 involving over 8,000 women showed that the women taking testosterone were more likely to report a benefit in their sex lives, with improved arousal, ability to have an orgasm and sexual well-being when compared to those taking a placebo.

Current guidance states that testosterone can be considered for low sexual desire if HRT alone is not effective and if other causes (e.g. relationship issues or side effects of medication) have been excluded. In 2016, the British Menopause Society stated that this could be extended to include fatigue (see page 236).

Previously testosterone patches or implants were available, but these have been withdrawn from the market in the UK. However, the reasons for this were not related to any safety issues, rather commercial ones. The safety data from when they were on the market is still available. As such, although testosterone creams are available in the UK, they are not licensed for use in HRT (they are given for other conditions), though doctors can and do prescribe them. Currently testosterone is only given to women who are already taking oestrogen in HRT.

Generally testosterone is given as a cream or a gel. You rub it into the clean, dry skin of the tummy or thighs, and the hormone is absorbed through the skin to increase your levels. Your doctor may increase or decrease the dose as needed.

AndroFeme is a brand licensed in Australia which is imported under a special licence to the UK. It is made with almond oil, so may not be suitable for those with almond allergies and is currently only available on private prescription (not through the NHS). If you are prescribed AndroFeme, use the enclosed applicator to measure out the dose. The applicator looks like a syringe and is marked so that you can measure in units of 0.5 ml accurately. Once you put the applicator onto the nozzle of the AndroFeme tube, turn the tube with the applicator on upside down (gravity helps!) and slowly pull the plunger of the applicator at the same time as you squeeze the tube of cream. As you do this, cream will fill the applicator syringe, which you can fill to the required amount.

Other testosterone gels include Testim and Testogel; these come with a screw cap or in sachets and you will be advised how much to use.

Apply the cream to the outer thighs or lower torso and massage in until it is fully absorbed, which takes approximately 30 seconds. Don't use other creams on the area as these can interfere with absorption, and keep the area dry for approximately one hour after application. To decrease the risk of developing dark hairs on the skin where the cream is applied, vary the spot where you rub it in. Avoid touching other people with the affected area until the cream is dry. As with any medicated ointment, cream or gel, wash your hands after applying.

Currently there is somewhat of a postcode lottery regarding testosterone on the NHS in the UK. In some areas, patients must be referred to a menopause clinic by a gynaecologist to receive the initial prescription of testosterone and then a GP can take over prescribing. In other areas, a GP can both initiate and continue prescribing testosterone. Campaigners are pushing for a national list of approved medications for HRT prescribing so that accessibility is improved.

*"For me, it was like, I'M BA–ACK!! Not just about sex, though good God I was glad to have it back, and to love it again, but I just recognized myself again, it gave me back my oomph – in all ways!"*

Alex, 53

## Does it work?

The answer is not a simple "yes" or "no". It can take a while for the hormone levels to rise and for symptoms to improve, but in clinical trials two thirds of women using testosterone reported an improvement in their symptoms as compared to a third of patients taking a placebo. So it doesn't work for everyone. Sex drive is complicated – low testosterone may not be the only issue, so fixing it may not solve the problem. But for many women it is effective, giving back not only their sex life, but a general sense of well-being.

## How long do I use it for?

It can take 8–12 weeks to see an effect with testosterone so it is recommended that at least a three-month trial is given. If there is no improvement after six months then you will be advised to stop. But if it is working you can continue as long as is needed, there is no arbitrary end point as long as any risks vs benefits are discussed and understood.

## What about side effects?

If you are replacing low levels of testosterone and bringing the levels up to normal there aren't likely to be significant side effects. Some women find hair growth where you rub the cream in; regularly moving where you rub it in can help.

If too much is given side effects such as acne, excess facial hair, hair loss on the scalp and voice deepening (rarely) can occur. Because of this your GP is likely to arrange blood monitoring tests to ensure you are on the correct dosage. If the levels are within the female physiological range, i.e. the expected range, then side effects are less likely.

**Can anyone use testosterone?**

There are certain situations in which testosterone should not be used, or should be used with caution:

◆ During pregnancy or breastfeeding – less likely if you are reading this book!

◆ If you have active liver disease or are a competitive athlete.

◆ Caution should be taken if you have a history of hormone-sensitive breast cancer – however, in discussion with your oncologists sometimes this is used depending on the particular hormone sensitivities involved.

---

An alternative to testosterone is to use tibolone, a synthetic form of HRT which contains oestrogen, progesterone and testosterone all together. For more information on tibolone please see page 239.

---

# Vaginal dryness

*"I did try to keep having sex, but the pain was awful, a sort of burning pain with every stroke. We had to stop, and now I am frightened to try again."*

Annie, 59

*"I couldn't even tolerate a finger inside my vagina, never mind anything else!"*

Maura, 54

Vaginal dryness is hugely common and often extremely distressing. It can occur at any point in your life, but is far more common after the menopause, with as many as four out of five women affected. Dryness itself is a symptom of what many doctors call vaginal atrophy (or atrophic vaginitis), but as the changes don't just affect the vagina, but the vulva (the external genitals including the labia and clitoris) and the urinary tract, a relatively new term has been coined: "genitourinary syndrome of the menopause" (GSM). However, for ease of reference in this book, urinary symptoms are covered in Chapter 5.

Vaginal dryness and its impact is seemingly the least talked about of all subjects related to the menopause, which in itself is still a taboo! Or perhaps it is not vaginal dryness which is the issue, rather the discussion of vaginas and sex in older women, especially after the menopause, which is the issue. Studies have shown that although 80% of women are affected by vaginal dryness, and about 60% report painful sex, 80% would not voluntarily discuss this with their doctor. There is a role to play for the doctor here: we need to ask the relevant questions, but the more that we talk about these issues, hopefully the more comfortable women will be coming forward to ask for help. And there are plenty of things that you can do and that are available over the counter as well.

*"It isn't just about sex, it is the whole time, I am just so, so itchy. And it isn't like scratching your elbow, you can't sit on the bus and scratch your bits can you?"*

Isobel, 59

◆ Dryness/soreness/burning/discomfort. The vulva may look red and inflamed. It doesn't always; in fact, the skin of the vulva and vagina can also look very pale and dry. There may also be some pain on passing urine as the urine touches the vulva.

◆ Painful sex. The medical word for painful sex is dyspareunia, which can be superficial (on the outside and in the vagina) or deep (in the pelvis/tummy). Here, the pain is felt in the vagina itself, often on penetration, and it is also often described as friction, or a burning-like pain.

◆ Itching. The dryness leads to itching, but scratching worsens the situation. It is easy to set up an "itch-scratch" cycle, where the more you itch, the more you scratch, so the more you itch. Itching is not only uncomfortable and irritating but the resulting constant shifting in your seat, fidgeting to relieve the itch (which is the same as scratching, so don't!), or scratching, can be embarrassing. The skin of the vagina and vulva is more fragile than before so scratching can lead to bleeding.

◆ Discharge. Although there are fewer secretions from the vagina after the menopause, in GSM there may be some discharge, often clear, white or yellow. This can be related to infection, which is more likely if the discharge is offensive in smell.

❖ Urinary/bladder symptoms – including urgency (needing to go to the toilet, now!), frequency and urinary tract infections. For more information on urinary problems related to GSM and the menopause please see Chapter 5.

All of these symptoms can be related to GSM, but they can be related to other conditions as well; for example, there are various skin conditions of the vulva, or more rarely, vulval cancer, so please do see your doctor.

*"Scratching didn't help, I just got more and more itchy. The only relief I felt was when I took a can of Coke from the fridge and used it like an ice pack between my thighs!"*

Niamh, 60

## Why?

*"I am amazed by how varied my symptoms are. I thought my periods would stop and I would get flushes for a while and then that would be that. I didn't know that I would be struggling years later with things still related to the menopause."*

Catherine, 65

The changes of GSM do not always occur straight away. While you can have hot flushes or memory problems, joint pains, exhaustion and any of a myriad of symptoms even before your periods stop, GSM doesn't tend to occur until a few years after. It often comes on much more gradually and much slower as it is related to the response of the tissues to the lack of oestrogen over time.

There are receptors for oestrogen all over the body, including the vagina, the vulva, the bladder, the urethra and the pelvic floor (essentially your urinary tract and your genitals). Over time, as the levels of oestrogen decrease after the menopause, the mucosa, or tissues, of the vagina loses their elasticity, and therefore the capacity to stretch during sex, becoming more fragile, and the vagina itself can get smaller. The vagina becomes drier and is less able to produce secretions and discharge; ordinarily during arousal and sex, the vagina produces more secretions and if it can't then sex can become painful. There is also a change in the pH level of the vagina, making it less acidic, and less glycogen is produced by the vagina. Prior to the menopause, the higher levels of oestrogen lead to high levels of glycogen, which encourages protective bacteria in the vagina. These changes change the bacterial and fungal flora of the vagina, making infections, including urinary tract infections, more likely (for more information on urinary tract infections see page 135).

## What can I do?

◆ Stop any irritants – no matter your age, your vagina does not need washing, douching, or even a spray of water up it with the shower. Your vagina is self-cleaning! The vulva, the external genitals, can and should be washed, but again use water, emollient creams or non-perfumed, non-allergenic soap (though the soap is not actually required). Pat dry after washing, don't rub!

- Wear cotton underwear, or at least underwear with a cotton gusset. Try to avoid wearing tight trousers or leggings with knickers and tights or, if you do wear these, then when you get home, take a few layers off. And your mother was right, consider going to bed without knickers!
- Change into fresh underwear after swimming, so avoid sunbathing in a wet swimsuit!
- Make sure your toilet paper and, if you are still using them, any sanitary products are not scented.
- It is possible to buy products targeted at vaginal itching or soreness which contain local anaesthetics. These are not recommended as they can cause contact dermatitis – inflammation of the skin – on the vulva. And they are covering up symptoms as opposed to treating them.

## Lubricants

*"I knew I was dry, so we tried different things including KY jelly, I mean that is the name everyone has heard of, right, so I bought it. It didn't help me at all."*

Laura, 60

- Lubricants – for use during sex. After all, if the vagina won't get moist, then let's put the moisture in the vagina. Lubricants are not vaginal moisturizers, they are only used during sex.
- Most sexual lubricants are not great for the skin of the vulva and vagina; in fact, lubricants containing glycerine and glycols can further irritate the vulva and vagina and those with a high pH can increase the risk of vaginal infections. Others may contain parabens, which some people prefer to avoid, or are petroleum-

based. Any lubricants that are perfumed should also be avoided. As a start, look for something pH-balanced.

◆ The other thing to consider is the type of lubricant. Options include water-based, oil-based and silicone-based. They feel slightly different, so it is a matter of personal preference. Water-based lubricants feel silky and similar to natural lubrication, but they don't last particularly long. Silicone-based lubricants are extremely slippery and are more likely to stain sheets. The latter also can't be used with silicone sex toys as they can break down the rubber over time. Oil-based lubricants are richer and creamier and last longer; however, oil-based lubricants are not appropriate if you use condoms as they can affect the integrity of the condom itself – not ideal!

◆ As looking for a pH-balanced, hypoallergenic, glycerine-free, etc. lubricant is not that easy, I normally recommend the following brands: Yes, Sutil or Sylk lubricants. Check the ingredients in case you are allergic to them; for example, some lubricants may contain nut oils.

◆ The double glide effect. While some may prefer a water-based and others an oil-based lubricant based on feel, silkiness and slipperiness, using a combination of the two creates what is known as the "double glide" effect and the Yes brand sells both, without any other ingredients which could be irritants. Oil and water don't mix so the oil lubricant slides over the water-based one, which can really help. You can put the oil-based lubricant on followed by the water-based, or one on you internally and the other on your partner/a sex toy. Try it!

## Vaginal moisturizers

◆ Vaginal moisturizers are different to lubricants in that while lubricants are only used for sex, vaginal moisturizers are used more regularly to moisturize the genitals. So if you have itching, general burning, soreness or discomfort you may benefit from a vaginal moisturizer.

◆ They can be used alone or in combination with lubricants; you may find you don't need a lubricant when using one, or need less, but they are fine to use together.

◆ Again, avoiding irritants and chemicals that can cause problems is the aim, as well as using a moisturizer with the correct osmolality – this means that it is similar to vaginal and vulval tissues and so will rehydrate them if needed without pulling moisture out or forcing moisture in, which can damage the fragile tissues.

◆ I usually recommend Yes vaginal moisturizer. Some moisturizers come with applicators and some without and are available on prescription as well as over the counter. Start off by using them daily and then after a week or two you can decrease to using them every three days.

◆ It can take three to four weeks to see an effect.

*"Oh the relief when we tried Yes was huge! And the pleasure too! It finally felt good again. No, better than good, it was great and just like that, without worrying about it hurting and actually enjoying it, I started wanting it more and more. My husband can't believe his luck!"*

Zoe, 63

## Topical oestrogen

*"I don't know why I waited so long before using the oestrogen, I suppose I had heard lots of bad things about HRT and thought it was the same. But I won't look back now, apart from to say I feel like I have the vagina of a 20-year-old again!"*

Tara, 65

Topical oestrogen is oestrogen which is given straight into the vagina and is a very effective form of treatment for GSM, not just for vaginal dryness or painful sex, but also for urinary symptoms. It is technically a form of hormone replacement, but it is not whole body, or systemic HRT because so little is absorbed into the bloodstream, it has no effects on the rest of the body (no systemic effects) and is considered to be virtually risk-free.

Vaginal or topical oestrogen can be given in combination with other HRT if needed. If you are taking HRT, not topical oestrogen, then if you have a womb you must take progesterone along with oestrogen to prevent womb cancer as the oestrogen alone can stimulate the lining of the womb to proliferate. However, this is NOT the case for vaginal oestrogen as there is no effect on the lining of the womb (for more information on HRT and womb cancer please see page 263).

Previously if you have had breast cancer then it was thought that you could not have topical oestrogen, but current evidence is that it is generally safe to do so. The only contraindication (reason to not give a treatment) for giving vaginal oestrogen is active treatment for breast cancer, not that you have had a past history of breast cancer.

Vaginal oestrogen does not increase your risk of breast cancer, nor does it increase your risk of breast cancer recurrence if you have previously had breast cancer. If you are taking tamoxifen or other treatments after breast cancer treatment, your doctor may ask for advice from your oncologist. Unless there is treatment for active breast cancer, it is generally considered fine and safe.

Vaginal oestrogen can be delivered in a cream, using an applicator, in a small gel pessary which is inserted into the vagina or a vaginal ring:

- The cream or pessary is generally used every night for two weeks and then twice per week. However, experts have said recently that the twice weekly dose may not be sufficient for symptom control and that it is safe to use on alternate days, or five days per week. Many women prefer the pessary as it is slightly less messy than the cream, or use a panty liner the day after they insert the cream.

- Vaginal oestrogen ring – an Estring. This is a flexible ring which is placed into the vagina and changed every three months, either by a healthcare professional, or by yourself. It can be left in during sex or removed and replaced afterwards.

- At the time of writing, it was announced that vaginal oestrogen, in the form of 10 mcg oestradiol tablets (named Gina), would be made available over the counter after a consultation with a pharmacist from September 2022. This would be without prescription for women over the age of 50 who haven't had a period for a year. Similar topical vaginal prescriptions would still be available via your GP.

There is no time limit for how long you can use topical oestrogen. Put simply, topical oestrogen works. It is safe and very effective, without significant risks. If lubricants and vaginal moisturizers are not enough, please see your GP as vaginal oestrogen works!

*"It changed my life, not just my sex life, but my life. No more itching, no more painful sex, no more burning. Just back to how it was 30 years ago. You couldn't pay me to stop, I was so relieved to hear I can be on it forever!"*

Natalie, 62

The short- and long-term safety of topical vaginal oestrogen, and its ability to treat genitourinary syndrome of the menopause, is clear.

Some 80% of women who have been through the menopause have some degree of genitourinary syndrome of the menopause, most commonly vaginal dryness, but other symptoms include painful sex, recurrent urinary tract infections and other urinary symptoms (see page 135). Having vaginal oestrogen available over the counter will potentially improve access for many women who need the treatment but, for various reasons, find it difficult to go to the doctor.

Topical vaginal oestrogen will not treat all the symptoms of the perimenopause and menopause, but it can be hugely beneficial for those with genitourinary syndromes. Improving access by making it an over-the-counter medication will be a positive step. Many of my patients describe vaginal oestrogen as a "game changer" in terms of their symptoms. As a treatment without long-term risks, it can indeed be considered a "life changer".

## Hormone replacement therapy

Systemic (whole body) HRT, be it by tablets, patches or gels, is also effective for treating GSM, though it can take a few months to notice the full effect. Or you may need to use both topical and systemic HRT togther. For more information on HRT please see Chapter 11.

## Other treatments

- Laser therapy – works to improve the blood supply to the vagina, stimulating healing and improving the quality and elasticity of the tissues.
- Ospemifene – an oral medication which seems to improve symptoms. It acts on oestrogen receptors to act as oestrogen in the vagina, but it does not involve hormones at all! It is generally only offered if vaginal oestrogen is not suitable, for example if you are having active treatment for breast cancer.
- Vaginal pessaries (brand name Intrarosa) containing the hormone DHEA (dehydroepiandrosterone), which is a precursor of sex hormones, are also available and can be effective.

# Problems with pelvic muscle tension

Pain may not be just due to vaginal dryness, but there can be an issue with the pelvic muscles. If the pelvic floor becomes weak and you are leaking, this may lead to a cycle of you holding and tensing the muscles continuously. Alternatively, part of the pelvic floor may have gone into spasm. Either can make the vagina feel too tight and so sex can be painful. A women's health physiotherapist may be able to help in these situations.

Alternatively, the pelvic floor can be too weak and the vagina may feel bigger than before, so you may feel less during sex. Regularly performing pelvic floor exercises can also help with arousal and with stronger orgasms. For more information about pelvic floor exercises and how to do them, see page 123.

# Sex toys, dilators and the menopause

*"Who'd have thought it, me looking at a sex shop online – there is a whole new world out there!"*

Katie, 64

I told you things would get interesting!

Penetrative sex is not always the be-all and end-all of sex for women, in fact most women cannot reach orgasm from penetrative sex alone. Non-penetrative sex can and does play an important role in many people's sex lives and relationships.

My patients are often surprised when I mention sex toys and dilators, but these can have a really useful role in helping you with your sex life! Using sex toys such as vibrators is associated not only with improved sexual function, but research showed that they are also associated with improved sleep, reduced pain and reduced stress, so worth a go! The vagina can get smaller after the menopause and less elastic and so it is more difficult for it to stretch during sex, be it penetration with a penis, sex toy or finger. There is also often an element of vaginismus, an involuntary tightening of the muscles of the vagina, making penetration more difficult; if, for example, you subconsciously are anxious about potential pain, you involuntarily tighten the muscles of the vagina. Using dilators can help with this – as long as the skin and mucosa are of a good enough quality to tolerate them, so lubricants, moisturizers and topical oestrogen may be needed. Vibrators can increase blood flow to the vaginal area so actually can help improve an underlying condition relating to vaginal dryness, as well as improving symptoms.

◆ Choose a "skin-safe" sex toy, made from silicone, metal, toughened glass or a particular plastic (ABS plastic) and not rubber, latex or jelly which can degrade or cause allergies.

◆ Use with an oil- or water-based lubricant such as Yes lubricant and be sure to clean after use.

## Dilators

◆ A dilator is a small device which is used to open the vagina. They come in varying sizes and you start with the smallest and work your way up.

◆ You use the dilators at home, gradually increasing the size. Using the dilator should be comfortable, and not painful.

◆ Lie on your back with your legs pulled up into a diamond shape. Use some lubricant and gently insert the dilator about halfway, aiming for the base of your spine (like putting in a tampon) leaving it in for a minute or so and repeat five or so times. You can also try gently pulling the dilator in and out and then gently rotating it to stretch the tissues.

◆ When you feel it isn't stretching any more you go to the next size up and keep going until you can comfortably tolerate a dilator that is just a bit bigger than your partner or sex toy.

- Once you are able to have sex comfortably, depending on how often you have sex you may need to keep using the dilator, for example if you have sex less than once per week.
- There are lots of dilators available online, but the rigid plastic models are less comfortable than the silicone variety, which feel more realistic.
- You can use dilators in conjunction with vibrators, such as an external clitoral stimulator, or use silicone dilators which contain vibrators or slim vibrators and then increase the size.
- Using a vibrator means that you also get some positive feedback in the dilating process – put simply it feels good, which makes you more likely to keep doing it, and helps you begin to associate penetration with pleasure again. It also can increase blood supply to the area.

But sex toys are not only to be used as dilators, they can also be used as part of your sex life. Orgasms can improve sleep and well-being and decrease stress levels, whether achieved solo or with a partner. Some women describe decreasing sexual sensation after the menopause. Put simply, sex doesn't feel as good as it used to and it may take longer to reach orgasm, or your orgasm may become ever more elusive. Using vibrators can help stimulate you and help you reach orgasm.

*"I had always used vibrators and toys as part of my sex life, but my girlfriend had not. It was opening up a new world!"*

Gita, 47

For those who haven't used a vibrator before, they are generally split into three types: external clitoral vibrators, internal vibrators or rabbit vibrators which combine the two.

- Using an external clitoral vibrator is often a good place to start, as the vibrations are stronger than the stimulation you can achieve manually or orally so may help if you have been feeling less than previously.

- Online stores such as Jo Divine or Sh! Women's Erotic Emporium are aimed at women and have lots of friendly and useful advice.

*"I am struggling a bit even to talk about it, but the truth is that I didn't masturbate very often and had never used a sex toy. My doctor advised me to try and somehow that gave me permission – if my doctor said so then I thought I should give it a go. I am so glad I did, I now realize that I didn't really know my body before and what I liked or disliked. Now I do and I can tell my husband, too. It has revolutionized our sex lives."*

Elsa, 59

## Psychosexual issues

Sex drive or libido is a complex issue, as we have discussed, involving both physical and psychological aspects which can be complicated and intertwined. If sex is not painful, and a physical cause of low libido is treated, it may be that there is a psychological component such as stress or anxiety. A lack of confidence in your postmenopausal body may lead you to not want to have sex, or there may be more deep-rooted issues about your self-esteem or your relationship.

*"I thought once the atrophy was treated and sex didn't hurt that it all would be fine, but it wasn't. We just seemed to have lost our connection and every time I made any move to be close physically, such as a kiss, he would take it as an invitation for sex, it felt like a lot of pressure."*

Pam, 63

A psychosexual counsellor may be able to help you reach an understanding of any issues, as well as giving you and your partner techniques to come back together. A commonly used technique to try to regain a physical connection is to actually take sex off the table! The stress and worry that any physical touch will lead to sex is taken away, then a period of time can be spent when you can only touch each other, or kiss and then slowly progress in time. By simply removing the pressure of penetrative sex, it may allow you to focus on the pleasurable sensations of other contact, building up in time, if you both want! Psychosexual services are available but limited on the NHS, they are also available privately.

So here we are, at the end of a chapter about sex, which starts with low libido and ends up with sex toys! But, if you want it to be, that can be your story too. There is help out there and although I appreciate it can be difficult to ask for advice and treatment, it really can make a difference.

*"I worried about empty nest syndrome, but quite frankly now I'm glad they aren't here all the time, since I got treatment our sex life literally has a new lease of life!"*

Melanie, 58

## SUMMARY POINTS

- Libido or sex drive is complex and can involve both physical and psychological aspects.
- Around the menopause many women report a decrease in their libido and/or a decrease in their sexual response – ability to be aroused or reach orgasm.
- Testosterone treatment as part of HRT can improve libido.
- Vaginal dryness is extremely common after the menopause and can lead to pain during sex.
- Options to manage this include lubricants, vaginal moisturizers and topical oestrogen treatments.
- Sex toys such as vibrators can be useful after the menopause (and before!).

# CHAPTER 8:

# SAFE SEX

———◆———

Now that your sex drive has hopefully improved and sex is more than just pain-free, it's comfortable and enjoyable (remember those pelvic floor exercises ladies!), we have to discuss safe sex!

On any day of the week I will be in my surgery asking women what contraception they are using and they will come up with a variety of reasons why they are not using any at all, ranging from their age to irregular periods or just not having thought about it! Unless you don't have ovaries or a womb, or you or your partner have been sterilized, the answer is you probably need contraception for longer than you thought. Not forever, but longer than you may have considered. And even after the risk of pregnancy has passed, you may still need to think about protection from STIs, in other words, using condoms.

## Why do I need to keep using contraception in my 40s?

Erm… you might get pregnant! And/or an STI!

I get it, you spend years worrying about not getting pregnant, then for many women there's a period of time worrying about getting pregnant (or not), and now you're back to worrying about not getting pregnant again. Women's fertility does begin to decline after the age of 35 and this decline speeds up after the age of 40 but the risk of pregnancy is still there. Even if you are having regular or irregular periods, flushes or any other menopausal symptoms, it does not mean that you can't conceive. Remember, during the perimenopause your hormone levels may be fluctuating wildly, and one month your ovaries may not be working but the next month they may well be, popping out an egg and leading to pregnancy! And even after the last period (and you can't tell it is the last period until you haven't had another for a year) there is still a risk of ovulation for a period of time afterwards and therefore of pregnancy. The risks of pregnancy itself, both to you and the baby, including miscarriage, increase with age.

Now if getting pregnant is OK, and you and your partner are content that there is this possibility if you don't use contraception, then of course that is up to you. But if getting pregnant is not ideal then you need to consider contraception.

## So how long do I need to use contraception for?

◆ If your last period was over a year ago (that is, you are postmenopausal) and you are over the age of 50, you will need to use contraception for one further year.

◆ If your last period was over a year ago and you are under the age of 50 you will need to use contraception for two further years.

◆ Once you hit the age of 55 contraception can be stopped as the risk of pregnancy is considered to be insignificant at this point.

◆ If you are on contraception which means that you don't have periods, then the advice is to use contraception until the age of 55, or, depending on the type of contraception, you can test to check if you are postmenopausal and then start counting from then.

◆ If you were diagnosed with an early menopause you will be advised to use contraception for longer – please see Chapter 3.

### Will it affect when I will go through the menopause?

No, contraception won't change when you go through the menopause but it might mask your symptoms. For example, contraception can affect your bleeding pattern. The combined oral contraceptive pill can be used as a form of HRT under the age of 50 because it can reduce symptoms (see page 187).

# So what can I use and why is it different as I get older?

For many women the contraceptive choices do not change. However, if your general health has changed some forms of contraception may be safer than others.

For each of the contraceptive methods I am about to describe I will give an effectiveness score stating perfect use and typical use. Perfect use is as it says on the tin, that the method is used perfectly, every time, no one forgets anything, nothing breaks, as if a robot were using the contraceptive method. Typical use gives an effectiveness score for what seems to be more usual, which is that we aren't perfect and mistakes happen! And although 90% seems high, remember that means that it fails on one in ten occasions! We do, though, have forms of contraception that are over 99% effective.

Remember, only condoms protect against sexually transmitted infections (STIs)!

## Short-acting forms of contraception

These are methods that you either need to think about on a daily basis, or even just as you are about to have sex.

### Male condoms

An oldie but a goodie. Condoms have been used for thousands of years. There are cave pictures and ancient Egyptian pictures of men wearing condoms! Rubber condoms were invented in the first half of the nineteenth century and have still come a long way since then.

**What is it?** A thin latex or plastic sheath worn over the penis as soon as it becomes erect as the pre-ejaculate contains a high proportion of sperm.

**How does it work?** Stops sperm entering the vagina and therefore meeting an egg.

**Effectiveness** – perfect use 98%, typical use 91%.

**Pros** – protects against STIs; no hormones.

**Cons** – can fall off or slip, need to remember them each time.

**Suitable for over 40s?** Yes.

**When can I stop it, for contraceptive purposes?** If no period for a year and you are under 50 then you can stop after two years; if over 50 then stop after one year. Or stop after age 55.

*"I didn't really think about it, periods went AWOL and so did the trusty pack of condoms I carried around. An unpleasant brush with chlamydia taught me otherwise!"*

Anne, 51

## Female condoms

**What is it?** A soft plastic sheath that is worn in the vagina.

**How does it work?** Stops sperm entering the vagina and meeting an egg.

**Effectiveness** – perfect use 95%, typical use 79% (we have more effective forms of contraception than this!).

**Pros** – protects against STIs, no hormones.

**Cons** – can fall off or slip, not widely available, need to remember them each time.

**Suitable for over 40s?** Yes.

**When can I stop it, for contraceptive purposes?** If no period for a year and you are under 50 then you can stop after two years; if over 50 then stop after one year. Or stop after age 55.

## Diaphragm/cervical cap

**What is it?** A small flexible latex or silicone cap which is covered in spermicide and put into the vagina to cover the cervix.

**How does it work?** The cervix is covered with the aim of stopping sperm from getting through; the spermicide kills sperm.

**Effectiveness** – perfect use 92–96%, typical use 71–88% (that means it doesn't work nearly three times out of ten!).

**Pros** – can be put in any time before sex (though more spermicide is needed after 3 hours); so you don't have to think about it just at the crucial moment; doesn't contain hormones.

**Cons** – doesn't protect against STIs; need to insert prior to sex and leave in for 6 hours afterwards; if you have sex multiple times you will need to leave the diaphragm in but insert more spermicide; you need to use the correct size (which may change, for example after childbirth).

**Suitable for over 40s?** Yes.

**When can I stop it, for contraceptive purposes?** If no period for a year and you are under 50 then you can stop after two years; if over 50 then stop after one year. Or stop after age 55.

*"I blame my mother, she used a diaphragm so I did too! It was a pleasant surprise to change to a coil, something I could forget about instead of faffing about, putting it in, taking it out."*

Laura, 49

## Combined oral contraceptive pill

**What is it?** Been around since the 1960s and is a pill containing both the hormones oestrogen and progesterone.

**How does it work?** Prevents ovulation; without an egg there can be no fertilization. Depending on how you take it you will have a withdrawal bleed "period", every month or less often. The combined oral contraceptive pill can be taken in a tailored way, including taking it continuously, without a break. If at some point you develop spotting for four days you then have a four-day break and then start again, so you actually may not bleed very often at all!

**Effectiveness** – perfect use over 99%, typical use around 91% (though this increases if you don't have a pill-free break each month).

**Pros** – can reduce period pain and heaviness of bleeding, may help with PMS and acne. The other main advantage of the combined pill is that the hormones it contains can be used as HRT in the under 50s – two birds with one stone! It also can help maintain bone mineral density and therefore decrease the risk of osteoporosis.

**Cons** – need to take daily and remember to start again after a pill-free break; severe diarrhoea or vomiting can decrease effectiveness. Side effects can include breast tenderness, or sometimes changes in mood, but changing the type of combined hormonal contraceptive pill you are on can often help with these.

**Suitable for over 40s?** Yes up to age 50. As long as you have no other risk factors or contraindications to use the combined pill, such as smoking over the age of 35, you can continue to use it until the age of 50, though your doctor may recommend a pill which contains a lower dose of oestrogen. After the age of 50 you will need to change to a different form of contraception as the risks of continuing after that point outweigh the benefit.

**When can I stop it, for contraceptive purposes?** If your periods stop under the age of 48, and you have no other contraindications to being on the pill, you can use it for the required two years after the menopause and finish by age 50. If you are going to be over 50 years old and still need contraception you will need an alternative method.

**Can you test me for the menopause while I am on it to see if I can stop?** No, the hormones interfere with any test, which isn't needed to diagnose the menopause but perhaps could be useful to help work out how long you need contraception for.

The contraceptive patch and contraceptive vaginal ring also contain both oestrogen and progesterone, the patch delivers the medication through the skin and the ring into the vagina. They work in the same way as the combined pill, and have the same effectiveness and can be used for the same period of time (until age 50). Their added benefit is that they don't need to be taken daily, instead can be changed every three weeks.

*"I have been happy on the pill, it controls my period pains and indeed when my periods come so I don't need to worry if I am going on holiday or something. So I was delighted to hear I could continue till 50 and that it may well treat any menopausal symptoms that otherwise may have been appearing."*

Ruth, 47

## Progesterone-only pill (POP)

**What is it?** A pill containing only progesterone. There are two forms: the older style mini pill which is taken daily and has to be taken in the same 3-hour window (lie-in or no lie-in), and a newer form (desogestrel), which has a 12-hour window to take it. There is no pill-free break with a progesterone-only pill.

**How does it work?** The progesterone works to make the mucous in the cervix very thick, so it is impenetrable to sperm. If the sperm can't get through, it can't fertilize an egg. Desogestrel is different to other POPs as it generally also stops ovulation.

**Effectiveness** – perfect use over 99%, typical use around 91%.

**Pros** – doesn't contain oestrogen, so if you have a contraindication to taking the combined pill such as a high body mass index or smoking in addition to being over 35 years old it can still be used.

**Cons** – needs to be taken daily, within a 3- or 12-hour window. The most common side effect is irregular bleeding though it can also cause acne and affect mood.

**Suitable for over 40s?** Yes, safe for use until age 55.

**When can I stop it, for contraceptive purposes?** If no period for a year and you are under 50, then you can stop after two years; if over 50 then stop after one year. Or stop after age 55.

**Can you test me for the menopause while I am on it to see if I can stop it?** YES! This is a form of hormonal contraception where we can! If you are over the age of 50, we can take a blood test for follicle-stimulating hormone (FSH). If the level is over 30 IU/mL you will be considered to be postmenopausal and can then stop taking contraception after a further year.

*"I know I am supposed to stop smoking, of course I do. But I also know I am not going to. I don't like the idea of something in me for a long time so am not keen on a coil, Cerazette works for me!"*

Cath, 46

## Long-acting forms of contraception

Probably the main advantage of a long-acting form of contraception is that you don't have to think about them for months or, with most of them, for years. No remembering to take pills, or wondering if you missed one, once they are in they are in. This means that there is no longer a difference between perfect use and typical use, there are no user errors to be made. And, just in case you do change your mind, they are reversible and can be removed.

## Contraceptive implant

**What is it?** The contraceptive implant is a small flexible rod, about the size of a hair grip, which is inserted under the skin of the inside of the upper arm and releases progesterone.

**How does it work?** The progesterone released by the implant makes the mucous in the cervix thick so no sperm can get through and can also prevent ovulation.

**Effectiveness** – perfect use over 99%, typical use over 99%.

**How long does it last?** Three years.

**Pros** – contains a smaller dose of progesterone than oral pills so less likely to have any side effects. Can remain in situ for three years.

**Cons** – can change your bleeding pattern, in that the bleeding can become irregular or may stop (though you may consider this a good thing!). More rarely the bleeding can become more prolonged. A small procedure is required to insert and remove the implant using local anaesthetic.

**Suitable for over 40s?** Yes, safe until age 55.

**When can I stop it, for contraceptive purposes?** If no period for a year and you are under 50, then you can stop after two years; if over 50 then stop after one year. Or stop after age 55.

**Can you test me for the menopause while I am on it to see if I can stop it?** YES! This is a form of contraception where we can! If you are over the age of 50, we can take a blood test for follicle-stimulating hormone (FSH). If the level is over 30 IU/mL you will be considered to be postmenopausal and can then stop taking contraception after a further year.

*"How's this for mother and daughter bonding? We both got our contraceptive implants together!"*

Helen, 48

### Contraceptive injection

**What is it?** This is an injection of progesterone.

**How does it work?** The progesterone released by the injection makes the mucous in the cervix thick so it is impenetrable to sperm. Can also prevent ovulation.

**How long does it last?** The injection needs to be given every 12 weeks.

**Effectiveness** – perfect use over 99%. Typical use around 94% (generally people leave it over 12 weeks between injections).

**Pros** – no need to think about contraception for 12 weeks at a time. Can lead to amenorrhoea – no periods at all.

**Cons** – can change the bleeding pattern to no bleeds at all (which I have also listed as a potential pro), irregular spotting or prolonged bleeding as well as changes to mood and libido, acne and breast tenderness. If used for long periods of time can increase the risk of osteoporosis. Requires an injection every 12 weeks, either in the GP surgery or with a newer system (Sayana Press) you can be taught to do it yourself at home. Can't be removed, so if you can't tolerate any side effects you still have to wait for it to wear off.

**Suitable for over 40s?** Yes and no. If there are no risk factors for osteoporosis it is safe to use until age 50, if there are risk factors it is only used until aged 40.

**When can I stop it, for contraceptive purposes?** It depends: if you have no risk factors regarding your bone density and osteoporosis, if you have your last period before age 48 you will be able to use it until age 50, which is the two years required after the last period. If you need to use contraception after the age of 50 a different form will be required.

**Can you test me for the menopause when I am on it to see if I can stop?** Yes and no. If the blood test is taken just after the injection is given, the high levels of progesterone can interfere with the test. Instead the test can be taken just before the next dose of the contraceptive injection is due.

*"To be honest it used to be a bit of a pain seeing the practice nurse every 12 weeks, but since I have started with Sayana Press I do it at home, easy as pie."*

Rachel, 46

### Intrauterine device (IUD) – copper coil

**What is it?** A copper coil is a small T- or anchor-shaped device made of plastic and copper which is inserted into the womb through the cervix.

**How does it work?** The copper makes the cervical mucous thick so sperm can't get through. It also stops any fertilized eggs from being implanted.

**Effectiveness** – perfect and typical use over 99%.

**How long does it last?** Depending on the device used, five or ten years, but if a ten-year IUD is inserted after the age of 40 it can remain in place and be used as contraception until you go through the menopause.

**Pros** – it lasts for years, no need to think about contraception at all. It contains no hormones.

**Cons** – it tends to make periods slightly longer and heavier. Requires a procedure to insert and remove.

**Suitable for over 40s?** Yes. Safe to use until age 55.

**When can I stop it, for contraceptive purposes?** If no period for a year and you are under 50, then you can stop after two years; if over 50 then stop after one year. Or stop after age 55.

**Can you test me for the menopause while I am on it to see if I can stop it?** No need, unless you have menopausal symptoms under the age of 45. There are no hormones in the copper coil so it won't affect how often you bleed, so we go back to our previous contraception rules: if you go through your last period under the age of 50 you need contraception for a further two years, if over the age of 50 for a further one year.

*"I had my coil inserted at age 42 and the joy is: that is it for me, no need to worry about contraception at all from now until my periods stop."*

Jayne, 47

## Intrauterine system (IUS)

**What is it?** A small T- or anchor-shaped plastic device is inserted into the womb and it releases progesterone.

**How does it work?** The device releases a small amount of progesterone each day, making the cervical mucous thick to prevent sperm from entering. It also makes the lining of the womb thin so nothing can implant and in some women prevents ovulation, though not in all women.

**How long does it last?** Depending on the device used, between three and five years. A Mirena IUS inserted over the age of 45 can be left in until age 55 if being used for contraception. However, if the Mirena IUS is being used as the progesterone component of HRT, for endometrial (womb) protection, it needs to be changed every five years (it is licensed for use in this way for four years, but the British Menopause Society and Faculty of Sexual and Reproductive Healthcare advise that the Mirena IUS can be used for five years as part of HRT).

**Effectiveness** – perfect and typical use over 99%.

**Pros** – lasts for years, no need to think about contraception. The Mirena IUS is also licensed for use as the progesterone component of HRT (note it is the only progesterone form of contraception which is). It contains the smallest dose of hormone of any of the hormone-containing forms of contraception. It is also licensed as a treatment for heavy menstrual bleeding, and by one year of use 90% of women have no bleeding with it at all.

**Cons** – requires a small procedure to insert and remove it. It can change the bleeding pattern, generally towards no bleeds by one year, but there can be irregular spotting, generally within the first three to six months. Occasionally there can be prolonged bleeding. The IUS contains the smallest amount of progesterone of any form of contraception as it acts locally, but like any progesterone can affect mood/libido as well as cause acne and weight gain.

**Suitable for over 40s?** Yes, yes, yes, this is a great choice for many women as it generally stops bleeding and can be used as the progesterone component of HRT.

**When can I stop it, for contraceptive purposes?** If you still have periods with an IUS, when you have no period for a year and you are under 50, then you can stop after two years; if over 50 then stop after one year. However, if you don't have periods with an IUS, as it can decrease/stop bleeding, you may need to test or stop after age 55. Even when not required for contraception, the IUS can be used for the progesterone part of HRT.

**Can you test me for the menopause while I am on it to see if I can stop it?** YES! If you are over the age of 50, we can take a blood test for follicle-stimulating hormone (FSH). If the level is over 30 IU/mL you will be considered to be postmenopausal and can then stop taking contraception after a further year.

*"I have always been plagued by heavy periods but as I approached the menopause they got entirely out of control, I felt I was bleeding more days than not. The Mirena coil (IUS) has sorted it out entirely. I don't bleed at all and when I got hot flushes my GP just gave me an oestrogen gel as well."*

Marion, 50

## Permanent forms of contraception

### Sterilization
**What is it?** In women the fallopian tubes, and in men the vas deferens (which carries the sperm) are cut, sealed off or blocked.

**Effectiveness** – failure rate in females one in 200, in males one in 2,000.

**Pros** – permanent.

**Cons** – permanent. Requires a procedure: vasectomy can be performed under local anaesthetic but female sterilization requires a general anaesthetic. May lead to chronic pain in males. Doesn't affect periods or menopausal symptoms in women.

**Suitable for over 40s?** If you are sure, yes.

*"My husband always assumed I would be sterilized after our last child was born, so I told him to get the snip! Surprisingly enough he wasn't that keen. I have a coil now, it lasts ten years, so I rarely think about contraception at all."*

Susan, 49

A word on the rhythm or natural method, checking your temperature or cervical mucous. It doesn't really work well, with typical effectiveness being about 76%. It means you can't have sex for many days of your cycle, and if your cycle becomes irregular it is even more difficult to work out when it is "safe" or not, making this method even less effective. And withdrawal is not an effective method either, there is sperm in the pre-ejaculate!

# Do I really need it? I am on HRT

Yes you do. HRT is not licensed as contraception, so you may well get pregnant even if you are taking it. And I understand that this sounds counterintuitive, but you can.

If you are using the combined oral contraceptive pill, the hormones may well work as HRT to alleviate any menopausal symptoms up until the age of 50 but it is a form of contraception as opposed to HRT, which is not.

If you are using the Mirena coil as contraception, it can be used as the progesterone part of HRT; however, no other progesterone-only form of contraception such as the implant, injection or pills can be used as progesterone in HRT.

All forms of progesterone-only contraception – pill, implant, injection or coil, as well as non-hormonal methods such as the copper coil or condoms – can be used alongside HRT.

If you are using HRT we cannot do a blood test to see if you are through the menopause as the hormones involved in HRT affect the test. So the options are to use another form of contraception alongside your HRT, or if suitable use the combined oral contraceptive pill as both your contraception and HRT.

## Oops, I had sex without contraception, now what?

Women over the age of 40 can use emergency contraception in the form of oral medication, either Levonelle or EllaOne, or a copper coil (IUD). The oral medications are available from pharmacies with or without a prescription or from your doctor.

# Sexually transmitted infections

*"I honestly never thought about it, once the risk of getting pregnant was over, it literally never occurred to me to think about STIs."*

Holly, 54

It seems reasonable in a way, that once pregnancy is no longer a possibility or a concern, to stop thinking about contraception. Over 80% of people between the ages of 50 and 90 are sexually active – why shouldn't they be? But to no longer think about contraception also means no longer thinking about protection against sexually transmitted infections (STIs). Add to this rising divorce rates, starting new relationships, better medication such as Viagra to allow active sex lives and the rates of STIs are rising. Nearly 15% of women and almost 10% of men between ages 50 and 70 have reported having three or more sexual partners in the past five years.

Between 2012 and 2017 the number of STIs in those over the age of 65 increased by 25% in women, and about 15% for men and between the ages of 45 and 64 increased by 7% in women and 9% in men. Potentially the numbers are actually even higher than this as it may be that older people are less likely to come forward for testing, perhaps due to embarrassment, or even not knowing that they are at increased risk. Interestingly, for the same time period, the number of STIs diagnosed in the under 45s fell by 8%. Sexually transmitted infections include chlamydia, gonorrhoea, herpes, genital warts, syphilis, HIV and more.

The only form of contraception that protects against sexually transmitted infection is a condom, with the male condom being more effective than the female condom. And remember that some STIs can be transmitted through oral sex, such as chlamydia and herpes, though a condom or dental dam can help prevent these. If you are in a relationship where you wish to stop using condoms then it is wise for both of you to attend a local sexual health clinic for testing and to only stop once you both have been told you are free of STIs. And even if you are using condoms, regular sexual health check-ups for infection are a good idea as not all STIs have symptoms.

The message is simple — even when there is no chance of pregnancy there is a risk of STIs, so use condoms!

*"My doctor was great, she sorted my vaginal dryness and when I said that sex was so much better than before, she replied to go and have fun, but don't forget the condom!"*

Iris, 61

## SUMMARY POINTS

- If you go through the menopause after the age of 50 you will need to use contraception for a further year.
- If you go through the menopause under the age of 50 you will need to continue to use contraception for a further two years.
- After the age of 55, there is no further need for contraception irrespective of when you went through the menopause.
- There are lots of choices available with regard to contraception around the time of the menopause. Please see your doctor to see what is most appropriate or suitable for you.
- A Mirena IUS is often a good option as it works not only as contraception, but also treats heavy periods and is licensed to be used as the progesterone component of HRT, meaning that you would therefore only need to take oestrogen.
- Only a condom protects you against sexually transmitted infections, so be safe!

# CHAPTER 9:

# HEALTH CONDITIONS
# AFTER THE MENOPAUSE

◆

A patient once described the menopause as falling off a cliff; that she knew she had no control over the car she was driving (her body) and that disaster was imminent but she had no way of stopping it. But importantly she said that she knew she would survive the fall but didn't know what life would be like afterwards. To be fair I have heard patients describe situations in a similar fashion, from pregnancy (after all, you know you are going to have a baby but just the how and what happens next are unknown), to cancer treatment and more. But it is important to look at what happens next in terms of the menopause in order to be aware of potential health conditions and how best to prevent or treat them.

*"I made it, out the other side, through the hot flushes, sweats and thoughts of losing my mind, but I thought that was it, I didn't realize that the effects of the menopause could continue."*

Shari, 69

The long-term effects of being in an oestrogen-deficient state impacts all parts of the body – from skin and hair to the genitals –

and these symptoms are covered in chapters 4, 5 and 6. This chapter is going to focus on the longer-term health conditions which may be related to the menopause as well as covering self-care and the screening programmes available after the age of 50.

# Osteoporosis

Osteoporosis is a condition in which the bones become thin and fragile, meaning that they are more likely to fracture, or break, sometimes even without a significant injury. We tend to think of our bones as solid and inert but actually they are living hives of industry, constantly being broken down and built up again. As you grow during childhood and puberty, the balance is towards the bones being built up, with maximum or peak bone density in the mid 20s. The balance between building up and breaking down then is approximately equal until the mid 30s when it then shifts again, but this time in favour of breaking down. This means that after this point the bones are becoming thinner, but this thinning speeds up after the menopause.

*"I thought osteoporosis was a disease of old people, little old ladies – I didn't realize that I could have it and not know anything about it."*

Maya, 63

## What causes osteoporosis?

Bone loss is part of getting older but women lose bone more rapidly in the first few years after the menopause, due to the loss of oestrogen. Bones are not static, rather they are continually being broken down and built up again. Oestrogen helps the body absorb calcium, which is needed to maintain bones; and it also has an effect on the bones themselves, by helping the cells which absorb bone to break down, so less oestrogen means that the cells which break down bone become more active. As oestrogen levels fall, this protection also falls and the bones can thin more rapidly, with the result that women can lose 20% of their bone mass within five to seven years of the menopause.

This means that women are more likely to have osteoporosis than men. It also means that women who have a premature menopause are more likely to develop osteoporosis, as the oestrogen levels drop earlier in life, unless they are treated with HRT.

Other risk factors include: having a family history of osteoporosis, having used high-dose oral steroids for long periods of time (to treat another condition) and having a low body mass index, for example if you have an eating disorder. A history of other conditions such as having an overactive thyroid or coeliac disease also increases your risk as does long-term use of progesterone contraceptive injections.

Lifestyle factors can also increase risk, such as smoking and heavy drinking of alcohol, lack of weight-bearing exercise and a diet insufficient in vitamin D and calcium.

## What are the symptoms?

Osteoporosis does not have any symptoms, until there is a fracture and at that point the symptoms are related to the fracture, often of the hip, spine and wrist. The pain of breaking a bone is not the only issue; fractures can really affect the quality of life and how independent you can be. In fact, hip fractures are associated with an increased risk of death. Pain can also become chronic after a fracture.

## How is osteoporosis diagnosed?

Doctors use assessment tools such as FRAX to calculate your risk of having a fracture in the next ten years. They also use the bone density scan – also called a DEXA scan (Dual Energy X-ray Absorptiometry), which measures bone density. It takes a few minutes and is painless; you simply lie on the X-ray table and a scanner is passed over you and the amount of X-rays absorbed by your body is calculated at particular points, generally the spine and hip. You do not have to have any injections or lie in an MRI tunnel during a DEXA scan. The results compare your bone density to those of a healthy young adult and calculate a T score.

◆ T score above -1 is normal.

◆ T score between -1 and -2.5 is a decreased bone density, but not at a level to be considered osteoporosis. This is called osteopenia and depending on the result your doctor will advise on treatment.

◆ T score below -2.5 is diagnostic of osteoporosis.

## How is it treated?

Treatment aims to increase bone density and therefore strengthen bones to prevent fractures. There are various medications available. Your doctor will use a combination of your age, your DEXA scan result and your fracture risk scores to assess the appropriate treatment for you.

◆ Bisphosphonates such as alendronic acid (alendronate) and risedronate slow down the rate of bone breakdown. They are generally taken once per week and you must take them with a full glass of water and remain sitting or standing for 30 minutes afterwards to prevent irritation of the oesophagus. They take time to work and are generally used for a period of five years before a repeat bone scan. Bisphosphonates seem to continue to have an effect for a few years after stopping taking them.

- Selective oestrogen receptor modulators (SERMs) – raloxifene, acts similarly to oestrogen on bone to increase bone density, but blocks oestrogen receptors in other parts of the body such as the womb and breasts. It is licensed to reduce the risk of spinal fractures if bisphosphonates are not working or are not suitable, but can cause hot flushes as a side effect.

- Calcium supplements – having enough calcium is essential to maintain your bones, i.e. 700 mg of calcium per day, which is generally absorbed from your diet. However, additional calcium in the form of supplements may be recommended in osteoporosis.

- Vitamin D supplements – vitamin D helps the body absorb calcium and is required for bone health. If you have osteoporosis you may be advised to take a daily supplement all year round. If you are taking calcium and vitamin D supplements as well as a bisphosphonate, you should not take the supplements on the day of the week you take your bisphosphonate.

- Other treatments include denosumab, a six-monthly injection of an antibody which slows down the rate that bone is broken down, therefore increasing bone density.

## But what about HRT?

*"I needed HRT because my symptoms were out of control, the protection against osteoporosis is just a welcome bonus!"*

Gita, 57

HRT does maintain bone density and therefore can reduce the risks of fractures. Despite this it isn't recommended as a first line treatment for osteoporosis, as its effects wear off when you stop taking it and due to the small risks associated with HRT. Those risks themselves may be more likely due to age, for example the risk of stroke, though this can be mitigated by giving the oestrogen through the skin (see Chapter 11 for more on the risks and benefits of HRT).

HRT is recommended to women who experience a premature menopause, under the age of 40, to protect their bones as they have a higher risk of osteoporosis. If you go through the menopause under the age of 45 and have other risk factors for osteoporosis you may also be recommended to have HRT, at least until the average age of the menopause.

But HRT does work here and so if you have menopausal symptoms you will get the added benefit of bone protection as well as symptom relief!

## What can I do to prevent and manage osteoporosis?

In an ideal world, we would be looking after our bones in order to prevent osteoporosis and maintain bone health from an early age, from puberty! After all, the stronger your bones are when you are young, and the greater the peak bone mass density you have in your mid 20s, the longer these bones are going to take to thin to levels that can cause problems. Although without a time machine we can't go back to being teenagers again – and I am not sure many of us would want to – there are still some things you can do to help maintain your bone density and prevent osteoporosis. These are likely to still be of benefit even if you have been diagnosed with osteoporosis.

*"I try to eat healthily and had cut out dairy, as I thought it contained too much fat, but my doctor explained why I needed to eat it, so back on the cheese it is for me, though a low-fat version."*

Punam, 57

## Diet

Aim to eat 700 mg of calcium each day, though you may be advised to increase this amount to 1,200 mg per day if you have been diagnosed with osteoporosis (which is why many patients are also given a calcium supplement). Don't worry about eating foods which add up to containing a little more one day and a little less another as this is about getting an average amount of 700 mg of calcium per day. The most calcium-rich foods are dairy products and you can reach your 700 mg per day by drinking about a pint of milk (think about how much you have in your tea/ coffee each day – it all adds up!). Choosing skimmed milk or low-fat dairy options do not really affect the calcium content and may help you keep to a healthy diet. Other calcium-rich foods include fish where the bones are eaten, such as sardines or whitebait, as well as tofu, green leafy vegetables (though you need to eat lots of them), dried fruit, and calcium-fortified bread. So, drink milk in your tea, have a yoghurt and plenty of green leafy veg and fortified bread and you are well on your way to meeting your target! Unless you are advised to take a calcium supplement it is not necessary to do so and high levels of calcium are linked to other health problems.

Vitamin D is required to help the body absorb calcium and magnesium from the intestines, which are needed for bones. It is mostly made via the skin through sun exposure, but this doesn't mean that you should bake in the sun all day, though truth be told it would be a little chilly here in the UK! However gradual exposure of 10–15 minutes per day will build up your vitamin D levels. Vitamin D is found in a few foods such as eggs, oily fish and fortified cereals. It is recommended that everyone in the UK takes a daily supplement of 10 mcg (400 IU) of vitamin D throughout the winter months, from October to the end of March each year.

## Exercise

Weight-bearing exercise has been proven to help prevent osteoporosis. Remember that your bones are constantly breaking down and remodelling. The impact of weight-bearing exercise encourages bones to become and stay strong. Ideally you should be doing weight-bearing exercise from a young age and then keep on going!

Weight-bearing exercise means what it sounds like: you have to be on your feet, so that you are holding your own body weight, or rather your bones are. It can be cardio- or strength-based but you have to be bearing weight, so swimming or aqua aerobics, where your body is supported by the water, and even rowing or cycling are not weight bearing.

But walking counts! Get walking, just so fast that you can have a conversation but not comfortably sing is enough to get your heart rate up to be beneficial for your heart health as well as your bones. Climbing stairs is also good!

Higher impact options for weight-bearing exercise range from running, skipping to aerobics, star jumps and sports such as tennis also count, anything where you are on your feet. Aim for 150 minutes of exercise per week, be that 30 minutes of aerobic exercise five times a week, or shorter bursts of 10 minutes at a time.

You should also aim to do strength- or resistance-based exercise on two days per week. Resistance work means you use your muscles against resistance, making them pull on the bones which then react and respond by becoming stronger. The stronger your muscles, the stronger the pull on the bones and then the stronger the bones become. The resistance can be from weights such as machines at the gym or in the park, using a resistance band, but also your own body weight, such as squats or push-ups.

*"So here I am, 58 and still doing star jumps and getting out my old skipping rope, just like I did when I was seven! I do them in the ad breaks on the television, my doctor says it all adds up!"*

Leora, 58

**Smoking and drinking**

Smoking is associated with an increased risk of osteoporosis, therefore not smoking, or stopping smoking, is beneficial. And not just for your bones, it decreases your cancer risk – for all cancers, not just lung cancer – and it improves your respiratory and cardiovascular health. For more information on smoking and stopping smoking please see page 119. Drinking more than 14 units of alcohol per week is associated with an increased risk of osteoporosis, so if you do drink alcohol, try to stay under this limit (for more information on alcohol and units please see page 115).

# The menopause and heart health

Cardiovascular disease is a term used to encompass any condition caused by narrowing of the blood vessels. It includes angina, heart attack (myocardial infarction), stroke and peripheral vascular disease. Cardiovascular disease is the leading cause of death in post-menopausal women in the UK, it being nine times more likely that a woman dies of cardiovascular disease than breast cancer. Cardiovascular disease affects both men and women, but men have higher rates at younger ages than women. After the menopause this gap shrinks and the risk of cardiovascular disease in women increases.

Oestrogen affects the entire body, which includes the heart and all your blood vessels. As levels fall after the menopause, the protective effect of oestrogen on the cardiovascular system is lost. Add to this an increase in weight and lack of exercise due to fatigue and joint pains means that lifestyle factors can further increase your risk of cardiovascular disease.

## What can I do to prevent heart disease?

◆ High blood pressure – medically this is known as hypertension and essentially means that the arteries have become stiffer and the heart needs to work harder to pump blood around the body. This increases your risk of cardiovascular disease, so if you have high blood pressure – often picked up after a blood pressure check at a GP surgery, or at the NHS health check (offered every five years) – treating your blood pressure to bring it down to a healthy level, be it with lifestyle changes and/or medication, will decrease your risk.

◆ High cholesterol – high cholesterol levels also increase your risk of cardiovascular disease, and these can be treated with lifestyle changes or medication.

◆ Diabetes – diabetes increases your risk of cardiovascular disease. Depending on the type of diabetes it can be treated with lifestyle changes and medication. Keeping blood sugar at a healthy level decreases the risk of cardiovascular disease.

◆ Healthy lifestyle factors including diet and exercise are all covered on pages 111-119 of Chapter 4.

## HRT and cardiovascular disease

The relationship between HRT and cardiovascular disease is complex. Originally it was thought that if cardiovascular disease rates increased after the menopause then replacing oestrogen with HRT would reduce the risk of cardiovascular disease. But initially this did not seem to be the case; in fact, the Women's Health Initiative trial showed an increased risk of cardiovascular disease with HRT, which then led to many women being taken off HRT or not starting. As discussed in the chapter on HRT (see Chapter 11), further analysis of the trial showed that it was those who took HRT over a decade after going through the menopause who had an increased risk and that this risk was small. Further research has shown that actually if HRT is taken within ten years of the menopause that it has no increased risk and may even decrease the risk of cardiovascular disease. HRT also improves symptoms such as fatigue, joint pains and insomnia, so you are more likely to keep exercising and therefore less likely to gain weight, again decreasing your risk.

## Cancer screening

The menopause does not cause cancer but getting older is associated with an increased risk of cancer and actually having a later menopause (after the age of 55) is associated with an increased risk of breast, ovarian and womb cancer. This is thought to be because more ovulatory cycles are associated with higher levels of oestrogen which affects the tissues of the breast and uterus.

The term "self-care" is heard a lot at the moment, followed by pictures on social media of lovely candlelit bubble baths, a bar of Dairy Milk and other treats and goodies to make us feel good. And while that is part of it, self-care is about looking after yourself and ensuring that your mind and body have what they need to be healthy. For some that may be eating kale salads and exercising but having occasional treats, for others it may be a pampering session, or some alone time, or just curling up with a good book. But for all of us it should include looking after your physical health. At its most basic level, self-care includes brushing your teeth and washing.

Self-checks and screening should also be included in this category of self-care, so look after yourself!

*"I have ignored my letters asking me to go for a smear for years. Who has the time?"*

Theresa, 53

## Breast cancer

Breast cancer is the commonest female cancer in the UK, with one in seven women being affected at some point in their lifetime. Regularly checking your breasts and attending the breast screening programme can help pick up any changes early, allowing treatment as early as possible, which has better outcomes.

### Examining your breasts

*"I never checked my breasts, but my partner noticed a lump when we were having sex — well, actually we then stopped having sex that time. But he knew my breasts better than I did myself."*

Michelle, 63

We need to check our breasts and we need to do it regularly. The exact method doesn't hugely matter as long as you have a good idea of what your own breasts feel like so you can notice if there is a difference. The method below is what is suggested, but if another way is more comfortable or you feel more confident with it, as long as you are feeling the entire breast, nipple, up to the collarbone and in the armpit, then keep going!

You may notice that your breasts feel different depending on where you are in your cycle if you are still having periods; for example, they often become more tender or lumpy before the period starts. After the menopause, the breasts tend to feel less firm. And it is totally normal to have breasts which are different sizes!

Before you start it is useful to know what you are looking for, but in a nutshell it is a change – that something is different about one of the breasts. For example:

- A change in the size or shape of a breast.
- A nipple becoming inverted – if you have always had inverted nipples this is not a change, it is only if this is new for you. Or if your nipple starts pointing in a different direction.
- Skin changes such as dimpling of the skin, so it looks like the surface of an orange (*peau d'orange*), or if an area of skin looks puckered, as if it is tethered to something underneath.
- A new lump – this can be one lump or an area full of little lumps and bumps that were not previously present.
- A thickening of an area of the breast.
- Nipple discharge, which can be bloodstained.
- New pain in one breast – breast pain is common in women, but tends to affect both breasts. Breast pain actually is rarely a symptom of breast cancer, but new onset of pain in one breast should be assessed.

So how do I do it? There aren't rights or wrongs to self-examination, just ensure you are covering the whole breast, starting as high as your collarbone and not forgetting your armpit. A suggested method:

- Start by standing in front of a mirror with your arms by your sides and look for any changes in the breasts. Then lift your arms above your head, or put them behind your head as if you are sunbathing and look again.
- Then examine each breast, leave one arm up behind your head and use the other to examine the opposite breast. You can do this standing up, sitting or lying down, but you may find it easiest to do in the shower or bath using a soapy hand as this can help your hand glide over the skin, but is not a requirement!
- You can imagine that each breast is a clock and work your way round the breast by running your hand from each number down to the nipple. But you don't have to use a particular method, as long as you feel the entire breast.
- Don't forget to check the areola, nipple and the armpit.

The next question which is asked is how often should I examine my breasts? Aim for monthly. If you are still having periods use them as a physical reminder to check your breasts after the period stops, as you may notice that your breasts are always slightly different before your period. If not, then set a date, such as the first of every month, and then perhaps an alarm on your phone to remind you.

*"I'm a good girl, always have been, and when I found out I was supposed to check my breasts I did so religiously every month. I am so glad that I did, as one month I found something. Because it was caught early it was removed, I had some radiotherapy and that was that."*

Rashmi, 61

If you do notice a change or find something which concerns you then please see your doctor as soon as possible. A change does not mean that you have breast cancer, but your GP will refer you on a two-week suspected cancer wait to be seen in a breast clinic at a local clinic. These tend to be "one-stop shops" where you see a breast specialist, are examined, have imaging such as an ultrasound and/or mammogram and then possibly have a tiny sample taken for biopsy with a needle (after using some local anaesthetic so you don't feel it!) all at the same clinic. This means that you don't keep on having to go back for tests and although it also means that you will spend most of a morning or afternoon at the clinic you will get a faster diagnosis. Depending on what is found and what tests are done you may be asked to return for the biopsy results a week or so later. But most changes in the breasts are benign – they can be due to a cyst, or other benign growth – so being referred does not mean that you have breast cancer, rather that you have a symptom which needs to be assessed.

The message is this, check your breasts, check regularly and check the whole breast and if you notice something that is different or concerns you see your doctor.

## Breast screening programme

The aim of the breast cancer screening programme in the UK is to detect breast cancer early, to allow early treatment, hopefully before the cancer has spread, so that treatment is more likely to be successful. The programme involves a mammogram, which is an X-ray of the breasts, and it may also pick up changes or even cancers of the breast which are unlikely to spread further.

Therefore it has the potential to lead to unnecessary investigations or even unnecessary treatment as well as causing anxiety about your condition. One in 25 women are called back for further investigation after having a screening mammogram, though this doesn't mean that there is cancer.

Everything in medicine is an assessment between potential risks and potential benefits. Let's add in some numbers – breast screening saves approximately one life out of every 200 women screened, saving about 1,300 lives from breast cancer in the UK annually. This has to be balanced against the fact that due to the screening programme, three per 1000 will be diagnosed with a cancer which not only would not have been found without screening but would never have become life-threatening. Over a year this means that some women in the UK are offered treatment that they potentially do not need, as the tumour would not have grown, spread or caused problems.

The overall balance is that due to screening 1,300 women's deaths will be prevented from breast cancer, but some women are diagnosed with a cancer which would not have caused death. So for every one woman whose life is saved, approximately three are diagnosed with cancer, which would not kill them, but treatment is generally offered.

Mammograms are X-rays and so involve radiation. Per 100,000 women screened every three years between 47 and 73, between one and ten extra cases of breast cancer will be caused from the radiation. The dose of radiation is one of the reasons why, unless you are at higher risk, you are offered a mammogram every three years instead of annually.

So the screening programme isn't perfect and more research is being done to try to find a method of discovering which breast cancers are likely to spread and become life-threatening and which are not. Research is also being carried out as to whether particular groups of women should have more frequent screening and others less; for example, women with denser breast tissue are more likely to develop cancer so perhaps should have more frequent screening than those with less dense breast tissue.

*"There was lots in the paper about the screening programme not working, women not being called or not being told their results, but the bottom line for me is this, it might stop me dying from breast cancer, so I always go."*

Sarah, 59

Currently this is the programme that we have, and while it isn't perfect, it picks up more than 18,000 cases of breast cancer (often at early stages) per year in the UK. Out of these, it prevents 1,300 deaths from breast cancer per year. So when it is my turn, I will be going.

## How often?

You will be invited for breast screening every three years between the ages of 50 and 70. After the age of 70 you are still eligible to have the screening test every three years, though you won't automatically be invited to do so. Instead you will have to contact your local screening centre to arrange it.

If you are thought to be at higher risk of breast cancer, for example due to your family history, your doctor may refer you to a genetic clinic to assess whether you should be offered annual mammogram screening from your 40s. Depending on your risk and if you carry particular genetic mutations associated with breast cancer you may be offered annual MRI scans of the breasts from the age of 20 or 30.

## How is a mammogram done?

You will be asked to remove the top half of your clothes and your bra. One breast will be placed on the X-ray machine and then an X-ray plate placed on top. The breast is squeezed between the two plates. Two X-rays are then taken from different angles, and then the procedure is repeated on the other side\. As the breasts are compressed between the X-ray plates it can be slightly uncomfortable but it only lasts a few seconds. Small breasts or big, it is possible to carry out a mammogram! The results are generally received within two weeks, and remember for the majority of women these are normal and you will be called again in three years. One in 25 women will be recalled for further investigation but this doesn't mean you have cancer!

*"I have big breasts, a size G, but my friend is a double A. We always laugh about my huge breasts being squished at a mammogram but she says they always find something to squash at hers! Only lasts a few seconds and then see you in three years!"*

Kate, 58

## Cervical cancer

Cervical screening is unique to the screening programme because it picks up cancer before it exists. The test previously looked at the cells to check for changes, but this was changed to primary human papilloma virus (HPV) testing in England, Scotland, and Wales in 2019, with Northern Ireland aiming to follow by 2023. This means that although the process of taking the test is the same, the sample will be tested for high-risk HPV which is the virus that causes the majority of cases of cervical cancer. If high-risk HPV is found then the cells will be examined for changes that have the potential to turn into cancer if left untreated.

*"I do it but I hate it. I know I shouldn't be but I am embarrassed and it isn't pleasant, but each time I reward myself afterwards and am so glad that I have had it done!"*

Laura, 53

## How often?
In England and Northern Ireland you will have been invited to attend cervical screening every three years from the age of 25 but after 50 this becomes every five years until you are 64; in Scotland and Wales you will be invited every five years from age 25 to age 64. The screening programme stops at the age of 65, though if you have recently had an abnormal smear and have been advised to attend for follow-up you will still be invited for this, irrespective of your age. There are currently discussions about extending the cervical screening programme to the age of 75.

## What does the test involve?
The test involves a plastic speculum being inserted into the vagina, to hold the walls of the vagina away in order that the cervix can be

seen. A small brush is then used to collect some of the cells from the cervix. A smear test takes a few minutes and for many women causes no discomfort at all, some women say there is a stretching type of discomfort as the speculum is inserted and others that the brush collecting the cells from the cervix causes a momentary pain like period pain.

After the menopause, the skin of the vagina can become thinner and drier and the process of taking a smear test can become more painful. If that is the case then please do talk to your doctor, using a vaginal moisturizer in the lead up to the test (but not on the day itself) can be useful. Alternatively your doctor may consider giving a two-week course of oestrogen cream before the test in order to improve the quality of the skin and decrease any discomfort. If you are concerned about the test, please do make an appointment to speak to your doctor or nurse first, for example if you know that you are very affected by the process of having a test, or it is difficult for another reason, book a double appointment so you can have the time you need.

The test results should be sent to you within two weeks. For most women the results will be normal but if not you may be required to either re-attend earlier than expected or be invited to have a colposcopy, where a special microscope is used to examine the cells of the cervix.

Currently there is a pilot study being carried out into self-sampling cervical screening which involves you inserting a swab (like a long cotton bud) into the vagina to take a sample to test for HPV. Only if that is positive would you be required to attend a more traditional smear test. Although this is at the testing stages, it could help more women have their cervical screening.

If you have symptoms which could be due to cervical cancer, such as bleeding in between your periods, or after sex, pelvic pain or an abnormal vaginal discharge, please see your doctor.

*"I had an 'inadequate' smear test which meant I had to go again earlier than expected and mentioned to my GP that I was scared as it had really hurt before. She gave me some vaginal oestrogen and it really helped, and helped sex too!"*

Chloe, 58

*"It isn't that I am embarrassed, or that it hurts, but I was assaulted years ago and find the process really difficult. What helps me is booking a double appointment so they can take their time and my friend comes for moral support."*

Laurel, 54

## Bowel cancer screening

Not directly related to the menopause or women's health, but colorectal screening is part of the screening programme and starts after the menopause. Colorectal or bowel cancer is a common form of cancer, affecting one in 20 people in the UK in their lifetimes. Early detection is more likely to lead to successful treatment, and screening often picks up bowel polyps, which are often benign, though can turn cancerous and so are removed. Bowel cancer screening is done via faecal immunochemical testing, which involves looking for hidden blood in your poo, and is offered every two years between 60 and 74, although the programme is gradually expanding to start from the age of 50.

## Other cancers for which there is no screening programme

There are many other conditions which do not have a screening programme at present. The following two are a common concern for women around the time of or after the menopause:

- Endometrial cancer – also known as womb or uterine cancer. If you have postmenopausal bleeding (bleeding after you have been through the menopause and not bled for one year) then please see your doctor for further investigation. Benign causes can include a thickening of the lining of the womb or a polyp, but you will have investigations to rule out endometrial cancer.

- Ovarian cancer – often described as a "hidden" cancer, as it can present with very non-specific symptoms which means that it often isn't detected in the early stages. Symptoms can include feeling bloated, abdominal or pelvic pain, feeling full earlier than previously, back pain, pain during sex and needing to go to the toilet more frequently. If you are concerned then please see your doctor.

## NHS health check

A health check is offered on the NHS between the ages of 40 and 74 every five years if you don't have particular health conditions such as heart disease or diabetes. You will be invited to see a nurse and have your body mass index checked (your height and weight), as well as your blood pressure and be given a blood test. The aim of the health check is to diagnose or assess your risk of heart disease, stroke, diabetes and kidney disease as well as giving advice on how to decrease your risk of developing these conditions.

*"I'm glad I went as finding out I had high blood pressure was the turning point for me, I went on to lose three stone!"*

Donna, 58

## SUMMARY POINTS

- Osteoporosis is a condition where the bones are thinner and more fragile. It is more common in women after the menopause.
- It is treated with various medications including bisphosphonates.
- HRT can be protective and help treat osteoporosis.
- Weight-bearing exercise can help maintain bone health.
- There is an increased risk of cardiovascular disease after the menopause, so this is a prime opportunity to look at any lifestyle factors such as smoking, exercise and diet.
- Women between 50 and 70 are offered three-yearly mammograms, and can request them three yearly after the age of 70.
- Women between 25 and 64 are offered cervical screening. In England and Northern Ireland this is currently every three years from 25 to 49 and then every five years between ages 50 and 64, while in Scotland and Wales it is every five years between the ages of 25 and 64.
- There is no specific screening programme currently for womb or ovarian cancer, but please see your doctor if you have bleeding more than one year after the menopause or if you have symptoms such as abdominal pain or persistent bloating.

# CHAPTER 10:

# WORKING 9-5: THE MENOPAUSE AND WORK

———◆———

Women work, sometimes because we have to, sometimes because we need to and sometimes because we want to! Over 70% of women between the ages of 16 and 64 are employed, compared with 53% in 1971. In fact, women have always worked, it is just that the type of work that they did, and indeed continue to do, was often at home and not paid. After all, raising a family (if that has been your choice) and running a household without sometimes wanting to kill one of the kids is a piece of cake, and not work at all, right? And if that situation doesn't describe you then you will have your own challenges I am sure. And the reward is… more work! More women are in the workplace than ever before, which is both brilliant and exhausting as they continue to shoulder most of the burden at home. Yes, I am generalizing here; no, I am not putting men down. I am simply stating facts. If the modern-day woman is supposed to have it all, they are also supposed to do it all, though perhaps that is a rant for another day.

# The impact of the menopause on work

There are approximately 5 million perimenopausal or menopausal working women in the UK. One in three people in the workplace is over the age of 50, and the State Pension age has risen to 66, meaning that issues around the menopause may become more pressing. That the menopause is a natural life event does not mean that it is always an easy process to go through. Of these women in the workforce 80% will have some symptoms and 25% can have severe symptoms. The symptoms of the menopause include tiredness and fatigue, insomnia, difficulties with memory and concentration — the so called "menopausal brain fog" — as well as anxiety, low mood and depression. These undoubtedly can affect your ability to function at work. The 2022 Fawcett Society report found that 44% of the over 4,000 women surveyed felt that their ability to carry out their jobs had been affected by their symptoms. Yet 80% of those surveyed had no support regarding the menopause in the workplace. Many women are anxious or embarrassed about speaking out and discussing potential difficulties with colleagues or their employer. There are various reasons for this: they might worry that they will be stigmatized for going through the menopause, that they will be considered "past it" in some way. Approximately four out of ten women surveyed in the Fawcett Society report said that symptoms have been treated as a joke by colleagues at work. They may also be concerned about how it will affect their colleagues' opinions about them, perhaps that it will impact on possible promotion or work assessment, or that they will be viewed as lacking, or changed in some way. Even more fundamentally, there are issues around a lack of understanding and awareness of employers, so that even if someone does speak up, their concerns may not be understood.

The impact of all this is that women are more likely to reduce their hours, turn down a promotion, change to a different role or even to leave work altogether, which can then have significant financial and other impacts on their lives. Research has found that 10% of women give up work, approximately 13% consider leaving work, and 14% reduce their hours due to their symptoms.

*"I used to pride myself on my ability to focus, zone everything else out, but for a few years I really struggled to concentrate. But I didn't dare say anything in case my boss decided to monitor my performance and may have said I wasn't doing as well as I should. I was worried I would lose my job!"*

Amy, 55

*"I left, I couldn't bear the constant anxiety, sleeplessness worrying about work and then the mortification of dripping with sweat whenever anyone approached me. It seemed better to leave."*

Shanice, 54

*"Why don't we talk about it? If we just spoke about it, perhaps I would have felt more supported at work. Instead I was too frightened to open my mouth, we don't speak about periods at work, why should I speak about not having periods?"*

Mae-Ling, 55

## Official guidance

The 2022 Fawcett Society study showed that approximately eight out of ten menopausal women reported that their workplace lacked support networks, absence policies and even information sharing.

There has been some progress, with more employers from various companies pledging to make workplaces more menopause-friendly. Some provide coaching and support, while others offer to cover the cost of NHS prescriptions for HRT.

It is recommended by the Faculty of Occupational Medicine that employers should be encouraged to create and follow guidance about supporting their staff during the menopause. The onus should not be on women themselves to raise awareness of the menopause, but for employers to be proactive. This guidance should contain information on the menopause: what it is and the symptoms which may be occurring as well as making employers aware that employees may find it difficult to speak about these issues. All staff should be informed about the menopause, even male staff, as although they won't go through the menopause themselves they may be affected by work relationships with women who are. It is particularly important that awareness of the menopause is raised among staff members who manage other staff. There should be an open environment, where women feel safe and confident to be able to discuss any work-based challenges related to the menopause.

*"My line manager is 20 years younger than me and a man, I have nothing against him as a boss, in fact I think he is good at what he does, but how can*

*I go and talk to him about why I am struggling at work, how could he possibly understand?"*

Jo, 54

It is the law that people should not be discriminated against on the basis of, among other aspects, gender, age and disability. Under the Equality Act of 2010 this would include women, of a certain age, going through the menopause! Cases have been won with relation to the menopause using this Act and in July 2022 a cross-party House of Commons Women and Equalities Committee called on the government to amend the Equality Act to introduce menopause as a protected characteristic. Currently, discriminating against people due to the menopause could be age, gender or disability related. It is not that the menopause is a disability, rather that the symptoms can have a significant and long-lasting effect on everyday activities and functioning. An understanding needs to be had that the impact of the menopause can last for months or years before and after the periods end. Employers also have a legal duty to ensure the safety and health of their staff, which again could include the menopause.

*"You may be able to go for a toilet break whenever you want in your job but I can't, I have to clock on and off every time I leave the floor and these are generally for scheduled breaks. My boss pulled me up in front of everyone for going to the toilet more than others. I am 58 years old, I don't need to be embarrassed like that."*

Farrah, 58

The Faculty of Occupational Medicine has produced guidance entitled "Guidance on menopause and the workplace" which may be useful for both employees and employers.

The following are suggestions as to what could be included in a work-based menopause policy:

- Information about the menopause and its symptoms, which could involve training, posters and other sources of information.
- Who to go to for information and support.
- Sufficient time to attend appointments.
- Sufficient breaks or allowances to ease menopausal symptoms such as stepping outside to cooler air, or to rest, or even sufficient toilet breaks.
- Physical alterations to the working environment: for example, allow a fan, or move a desk away from a radiator; and consider your dress code (if you have one) – is a uniform made of natural fibres, or can your employee, for example, take off their jacket?
- Flexible working for a period of time if required, such as changing hours or working from home for a few hours to avoid the heat and stuffiness of the rush-hour commute, or, on a more ad hoc basis, allowing someone to start a few hours later after a night of poor sleep.
- Who to contact for advice – both within the work organization itself (which could be HR or occupational health) and to advise women to seek support from healthcare professionals as required.

Why should we do this? Because the menopause will affect all the women in whatever organization they work for at some point, and if employers want to get the best out of them, to keep them at their most productive and useful, then they need to be supported through the menopause. A positive work place is more likely to be an effective one!

*"I know what I need, I need my team to know that I am doing my best, that things are tough for me right now but that I have started treatment and will be back to my normal self. It seems really personal to discuss it, but I need them to know."*

Alice, 51

*"If I could just start at 10 a.m. instead of 9 a.m., then I wouldn't be on the most busy train of the day, or I would even start at 8 a.m. to avoid it. The moment I step on the train the heat just overcomes me and by the time I get to work I am a mess and feel that everyone must notice that I look and feel so rubbish. I am happy to do the same amount of hours and I work as hard as ever, just starting one hour later would make such a difference to me every day. And yet, I don't know how I can say to my boss, erm please can I start a bit later as the train is too hot?"*

Micky, 54

*"I run a small business, employing seven staff and honestly I didn't think about how the menopause could affect my job until it happened to me. Once it did though I totally realized how much of an impact it could have. Now it is made clear to my staff that we are a menopause-friendly workplace, even something as small as someone being moved to being by the window can make such a huge difference to them, physically and mentally. And for me that means that they also stay being productive!"*

Kim, 58

*"Once I discussed my situation with my line manager, he asked me to give a presentation to all the managers about the menopause. They realized that they didn't know anything about it and felt that in order to help support their staff that they had to learn. Kudos to them!"*

Georgia, 56

*"At the time I felt I had no choice but to leave my job, but actually it turned out well for me as it meant I had the time to expand my coaching business. It is going really well and I always make sure to discuss the menopause."*

Dee, 58

*"Changes need to be made in big organizations, in big companies, to ensure that all women, including those not able to put themselves forward, are able to get the help that they need at work."*

Sharon, 57

## SUMMARY POINTS

- Many women find that their symptoms affect their ability to function at work.
- All workplaces should aim to have guidelines as to how to support women to continue to work through the menopause.
- Options include flexible working, being able to use a fan, or even more toilet breaks!

# Part Three

# HRT AND OTHER TREATMENTS

# CHAPTER 11:

# HRT – WHAT IS IT?

———◆———

HRT stands for hormone replacement therapy, and it does what it says on the tin – it replaces hormones that naturally fall to lower levels during and after the menopause. HRT can consist of oestrogen, progesterone and testosterone, and which hormones are used, or in what combination, will depend on your medical history and symptoms. This chapter will cover HRT, what it is, how it is delivered, risks, benefits, when to start, if you need to stop and much more.

## What is HRT?

Let's start at the very beginning, a very good place to start. When you read you begin with ABC, when you flush you begin with HRT!

### Oestrogen

It makes sense really, if most of the symptoms related to the menopause and beyond are due to reduced levels of oestrogen, replacing it should treat these symptoms!

◆ Body-identical oestrogens are generally used. This means that they have the same chemical structure as the oestrogens found in the body. There is currently a debate between body-identical vs bio-identical hormones, but in traditionally prescribed HRT body-identical oestrogens are used. For more information about body-identical vs bio-identical hormones please see page 283.

◆ Oestradiol is generally used, often processed from yams.

◆ It can be delivered by tablet, patch, gel, spray or implant. For more information read on.

If you have had a hysterectomy, whether or not the ovaries have been removed, you can have oestrogen-only HRT, i.e. no other hormones are required.

However, if you do have your womb you CANNOT have oestrogen-only HRT. Oestrogen stimulates the lining of the womb to build up (think back to our science lesson in Chapter 1), and without the opposing effect of progesterone this can increase the risk of endometrial or womb cancer.

## Progesterone

Progesterone is essential if you have a womb, to prevent build-up of the womb lining and prevent an increased risk of endometrial cancer.

◆ Again, there are body-identical forms of progesterone available, generally made from plants.

◆ Types of progesterone most body-identical include micronized progesterone, dydrogesterone, drospirenone and medroxyprogesterone.

◆ Alternatively, progesterone made from testosterone can be given, such as norethisterone, levonorgestrel and norgestrel.

◆ Can be delivered via an intrauterine system (a hormone-containing coil), tablets, patches or vaginal pessaries.

## Testosterone

The NICE guidance states that testosterone can be offered to women with low libido if HRT alone is not sufficient. This means that it is generally not offered as an initial treatment but can be if HRT is not sufficient. The British Menopause Society in 2016 recommended that it could also be offered to women with low libido and fatigue if these have not improved with HRT. Testosterone can be useful to help with libido, memory, concentration, fatigue and energy levels as well as maintaining muscle and bone strength and brain functioning. It is generally delivered through the skin with a cream. For more information on testosterone.

## Body-identical HRT

Body-identical HRT is that which is identical to the oestrogen and progesterone made naturally by the body. When compared to synthetic HRT, it is thought that body-identical HRT has lower risks of breast cancer, cardiovascular disease (heart attack and stroke) and blood clots. Body-identical HRT also seems to have fewer side effects such as fluid retention. Note that body-identical HRT (often also called regulated bio-identical HRT) is not the same as compounded bio-identical HRT – for more information please see page 283. Body-identical HRT includes various forms of transdermal oestrogen such as Oestrogel, as well as micronized progesterone (Uterogestan). A combined oral body-identical HRT recently became available in the UK, and is known as Bijuve. It is suitable for women who haven't had a period for a year, or who are over the age of 54.

## Can I start HRT if I am still having my periods?

Yes, you absolutely can have HRT if you are still having your periods. Whether they are coming monthly, irregularly, regularly or randomly, if you have symptoms you can have treatment. The type of HRT you are offered when you are still having periods will be different to that offered after your periods have stopped. Though, of course, nothing is quite so simple and there is a sort of halfway option also available. When you have periods you are offered what is called sequential HRT, when your periods stop, you are offered continuous combined HRT.

*"I didn't go to the doctor for years, I mean I still had my periods so I thought the doctor would say I had to wait for treatment."*

Suzanne, 50

# The different HRT regimes

*"Everyone has heard of paracetamol or amoxicillin, but those of my friends and I on HRT all seem to be on something slightly different! Some of us have periods, some of us don't and some of us seem to have chosen not to have them!"*

Isla, 52

HRT involves giving oestrogen to replace the low levels that are causing your symptoms. So oestrogen is always required. The progesterone component of HRT is only needed if you have your womb, in order to prevent the oestrogen stimulating the lining of the womb and increasing the risk of womb cancer. But when the progesterone is given will decide whether or not you still have periods while on HRT. These aren't true periods, but withdrawal bleeds from the hormones, similar to the withdrawal bleeds while on the combined oral contraceptive pill (though new guidance says that you don't actually need to have the break when taking the oral contraceptive pill, and therefore the withdrawal bleed, but can choose to take the packs back to back as part of tailored pill-taking if required: please discuss with your doctor before making any changes). Importantly, testosterone can be given no matter how the oestrogen and progesterone are delivered, be they sequential or continuous.

## Sequential HRT

Sequential HRT is used if treatment is needed during the perimenopause, when you are still having periods, regular or not. The ovaries are still functioning, though perhaps more sporadically, and sequential HRT will give a sort of "cycle". The reason to do this and to induce a regular withdrawal bleed is to stop irregular bleeding related to the still-working ovaries.

In sequential HRT you take oestrogen (in whatever form) daily and take the progesterone for 10–14 days each month. So the term sequential describes the sequence: oestrogen daily, progesterone for 10–14 days monthly. In the majority of women (approximately 85%) this cyclical progesterone will lead to a monthly withdrawal bleed.

There is a longer form of HRT, called long-cycle HRT, or Tridestra, where the oestrogen is taken daily but the progesterone is taken for 14 days every three months. This would then lead to a withdrawal bleed only once every three months. It isn't often used in the UK and the withdrawal bleed is often heavy with this regime.

If needed, for example to improve libido, you can add testosterone to sequential HRT. For further information about testosterone replacement see page 160.

## Continuous combined HRT

If your periods have stopped for over a year, you are considered to have gone through the menopause, the ovaries are no longer working. As such there is no need to induce a regular withdrawal bleed to prevent irregular bleeding. Continuous combined HRT is sometimes called period-free HRT.

In continuous combined HRT, both progesterone and oestrogen are taken daily. For the first six months there may be some irregular spotting, but after that point there should be no bleeding. And if there is please see your doctor.

Just like with sequential HRT, you can add testosterone if needed to continuous combined HRT.

Tibolone is a synthetic form of HRT containing oestrogen, progesterone and testosterone. This is sometimes chosen for women who have premature ovarian insufficiency as it combines all three hormones and is particularly good for bone protection. It is used for postmenopausal women as it is a form of continuous combined HRT. The risks and benefits of tibolone are the same as for other forms of HRT.

## The "halfway house"

The IUS, or Mirena, is a hormone-containing coil which is inserted through the vagina and cervix into the womb. It is licensed as a form of contraception (more info on page 149) for the treatment of heavy menstrual bleeding and also as the progesterone component of HRT, to protect the lining of the womb from the effects of oestrogen.

This means that you can have a Mirena inserted at any point, whether you have periods or not. With the progesterone part of HRT sorted, you can then have oestrogen daily either as a gel/patch/spray or tablet. Technically this is not a sequential form of HRT, as both are used together, but it is considered to be one as it is safe in the perimenopausal stage.

Advantages to having a Mirena coil and oestrogen as HRT:

- No bleeds. Or lighter, more irregular bleeds. Whether you were having periods or not, the IUS tends to stop or reduce bleeding, which is why it is also used as a treatment for heavy periods. For the first three to six months it can cause some irregular bleeding, generally light spotting, though more rarely heavier or continuous, and if this happens please see your doctor as treatments are available. By one year though, 90% of women will have no periods at all, and in the remaining 10% the periods tend to be lighter.

- It also works as contraception! Remember, contraception is still needed, for two years after the menopause if you went through it under the age of 50 and for one year if you go through the menopause after the age of 50. Contraception is required up until age 55.

- It decreases your risk of endometrial or womb cancer by almost 20%, more if you use the IUS for over ten years.

- It lasts for five years as both the progesterone part of HRT and as contraception, so you can have it inserted and then forget about it for a while! (Note other hormone-containing coils are available but are not licensed for HRT.)

◆ You can then have the oestrogen daily, in any form – tablet, patch or gel.

◆ As with other forms of HRT, testosterone can be added.

## When do you change from sequential HRT to continuous combined?

There is no right answer here, different guidelines say slightly different things! What we are aiming for is to switch over when the ovaries have stopped working, to reduce the risk of irregular bleeding. Some guidelines say you can try switching after one year on sequential HRT, or two, but most say that it is reasonable to change to continuous combined HRT after the age of 55. But let's be pragmatic, if you wish to change before, to try to avoid having periods, and then develop irregular bleeding on continuous combined HRT, you can switch back to sequential HRT for a period of time before trying again.

## Other HRT regimes

There are certain situations where a sequential or continuous combined regime may not be required, for example if you do not have a womb. Here, other HRT regimes are used, whereby only the required hormones are given.

### Oestrogen–only HRT

Oestrogen-only HRT is given if you don't have a uterus, and therefore do not need progesterone to stop a build-up of the lining of the womb. It can be delivered by tablet, patch or gel/spray and testosterone can be added if needed.

### Vaginal oestrogen

Although this replaces hormones it is not considered the same as taking HRT; in fact, using vaginal oestrogen for a year is the equivalent of taking one HRT tablet! It can be used alone or in combination with HRT. Commonly used brand names include Vagifem, Blissel and Ovestin. The only contraindication (reason to not give) vaginal oestrogen is active treatment for breast cancer. If you are on tamoxifen after initial breast cancer treatment, your GP is likely to discuss your case with your oncologist before prescribing vaginal oestrogen. Topical vaginal oestrogen is covered in more detail in the chapter on sex (for more information see page 172).

### Testosterone

Testosterone can be added to any of the above forms of HRT. For more information on testosterone replacement see page 160.

# How do you choose the right HRT regime for you?

As with any medication or treatment you and your doctor will go through a process of questions and decisions in order to decide the correct treatment plan, or in this case the correct HRT regime for you. Some of the questions to consider are as follows:

1.  **Do I need HRT?** Sounds obvious; if you didn't you wouldn't be here! But the symptoms you have will decide

on the treatment you need. For example, if you have flushes, joint pains, memory problems or any problem which affects the whole body in general you are likely to be recommended a form of HRT. But if you only have vaginal symptoms such as itching or painful sex, or urinary symptoms such as recurrent urinary tract infections without any other symptoms, you are likely to be offered vaginal (topical) oestrogen alone.

2.  **What is my past medical history?** HRT can be delivered in various ways, via tablets or through the skin with patches or gels. The way that the oestrogen in the HRT is delivered has different effects within the body, for example oestrogen delivered through the skin doesn't involve the oestrogen going through the liver, as it would do with an oral tablet. This means that the choice of how you deliver the oestrogen will have a different impact on issues such as clotting factors. So depending on your medical history, as well as a discussion about risks and side effects, you may be advised that it is safer or more appropriate to have the oestrogen delivered in a particular way. For example, oestrogen delivered through the skin in a patch, gel or cream has less clotting risk, so is the preferred option over oestrogen tablets in general. And remember if you don't have your womb, you can have just oestrogen alone.

3.  **Do you still have periods?** If you are in the perimenopause and still having periods you will need a sequential form of HRT. If your periods have already stopped you will need a continuous combined form of HRT – for more information see page 246.

4.  Do you still need contraception? HRT is not contraception and there is still a risk of pregnancy for two years if you go through the menopause under the age of 50 and for one year if you go through it after age 50, or until age 55, whichever is earliest. Up until age 50, as long as there are no contraindications, the combined oral contraceptive pill can be given as HRT. After this point, or if the pill can't be used for another reason, or if you would prefer not to take it, you will still need to use contraception. Choosing a Mirena IUS as the progesterone part of your HRT would cover you for contraception and then the oestrogen can be delivered via tablets/patches/vaginal ring. Progesterone-only forms of contraception and non-hormonal forms such as condoms and a copper coil can be used in combination with HRT.

5.  **What would you like?** Personal choice matters! It is your body and you must feel comfortable with the regime. For example, if you find it difficult to remember to take pills then another option will be preferable, but if you find the idea of patches abhorrent then do tell your doctor!

Below are some common names and preparations of the different HRT regimes to allow you to check what you are on. Not all the brand names are listed below, but I have included one or more of each of the main regimes.

## Oestrogen-only HRT

Only suitable for women without a uterus. Tablet form e.g. Elleste Solo (other oral brands available). Transdermal (through the skin) –

Evorel patch (other patches available such as Estradot), or Oestrogel or Sandrena gel, or Lenzetto spray. The initial choice of transdermal preparation is up to you, but some people seem to absorb the oestrogen better one way or another. You may opt for a gel or you may prefer a patch so that you don't have to remember it daily. Some women find that in higher doses the spray does not absorb as well, but this is not always the case.

## Sequential HRT

- Daily/continuous oestrogen – orally (such as Elleste Solo) or transdermally (such as Evorel patch or oestrogen gel/spray). Plus sequential progesterone, generally for two weeks each cycle. My preferred choice would be oestrogen transdermally plus Utrogestan for the progesterone component, as Utrogestan is micronized progesterone, which is most similar to the body's natural progesterone and is associated with the lowest risks.

- Oral oestrogen with sequential oral progesterone, e.g. Femoston tablets – depending on the strength, the colour of the tablets changes, but essentially the oestrogen-only tablet (generally white or red) daily, adding in the progesterone tablet (generally grey or yellow) on days 14–28. Then repeat without a break. The first cycle is started within five days of menstruation.

- Transdermal oestrogen with transdermal progesterone – e.g. Evorel Sequi patches (which contain oestrogen only) twice weekly for two weeks, then e.g. Evorel Conti (contains oestrogen and progesterone) twice weekly for two weeks.

Then repeat. The first cycle is started within five days of menstruation. Mirena IUS and transdermal oestrogen – via patch or gel. In this case, the Mirena IUS would also function as contraception if required.

◆ Long-cycle HRT – Tridestra as explained on page 238.

## Continuous combined HRT

◆ Daily oestrogen and progesterone – via patch or orally. Brands include Evorel Conti, or orally Elleste Duet or Kliofem. Taken daily without breaks. If changing from sequential to continuous combined, take at the end of the last scheduled bleed. The first and (at the time of writing) only existing oral body-identical combined HRT, named Bijuve, has recently become available in the UK (see page 236). It may not currently be offered nationwide on the NHS.

◆ Continuous oestrogen via patch (Evorel), gel or spray plus continuous daily oral progesterone such as Utrogestan.

◆ Mirena IUS and transdermal oestrogen – Evorel patch or Sandrena/Oestrogel gels or Lenzetto spray.

◆ Tibolone – a synthetic form of HRT. More information on page 239.

I appreciate that it looks daunting and complicated, but it doesn't have to be! Of course, you may not be prescribed one of the brand names above, or you may need to change brands.

# HRT – how do you use it?

It is likely that you generally know what to do if you are given a tablet to take, but how do you use patches/gels and sprays?

◆ **Where do you put the patch?** Apply the patch to the skin below the waist; generally the hips, outer thighs or bottom.

◆ **How do you remove the patch?** Simply peel it off. You may find that there is some residual sticky adhesive on the skin – you can wash this off or use a medical adhesive remover spray or wipe to help remove it.

◆ **What do you do if it falls off?** If a patch falls off then put on a new one. If you find that they aren't sticking well in general then changing brand may help, as may wiping the skin with an alcohol wipe or surgical spirit.

◆ **Can you shower/bathe/swim with the patch on?** Absolutely yes, the patches can be worn in water. They are safe for bathing, showering, exercising and swimming. As above, if you notice that one has come off then apply a new one.

◆ **Where do you put the gel/spray?** The instructions for the gels will give the licensed directions, which are to rub in the skin of your upper arm or on the inside of the thigh. You can also put it on your bottom, hips, thighs, tummy or lower back; just not on your breasts or genitals. The oestrogen spray is used on the inner part of the forearm. If you use more than one spray, spray the next dose onto a patch of skin next to the first region, not on top of it, or use the other arm. The inner thigh can also be used, but not the tummy or hips as this may affect absorption of the spray. Do not apply to the breasts or genitals.

◈ **Do you use all the gel/spray at the same time?** If you are using more than two pumps of Oestrogel, you may be advised to split the dose into morning and evening. The gel is not sticky or greasy; simply rub it in until it is absorbed. It doesn't tend to stain clothes. The spray does not need to be rubbed in; instead let it dry onto the skin for around 2 minutes.

◈ **Can you bathe or apply moisturizer straight away after the gel/spray?** It is advisable to wash or shower before the gel or spray. If this is not possible, wait at least an hour after rubbing it in/letting it dry. Also, wait an hour before applying any other creams.

◈ **Will my partner/child/pet get the medication if they touch my skin?** The gels rub in within a few minutes and the spray dries in about 2 minutes, but it is best to avoid letting others touch the area where you applied it for about an hour. Once rubbed in/left to dry it shouldn't stain clothes. Wash your hands after applying.

## SUMMARY POINTS

◈ If you have your uterus, you will need to take a combination of oestrogen and progesterone. If you don't have a uterus, you can use oestrogen alone.

◈ HRT can be started whenever it is needed, whether or not you have periods.

◈ Sequential HRT is generally given if the periods haven't stopped and it gives a withdrawal bleed.

◆ Continuous combined HRT is usually given when the periods have stopped and doesn't tend to lead to bleeding, although there can be spotting initially.

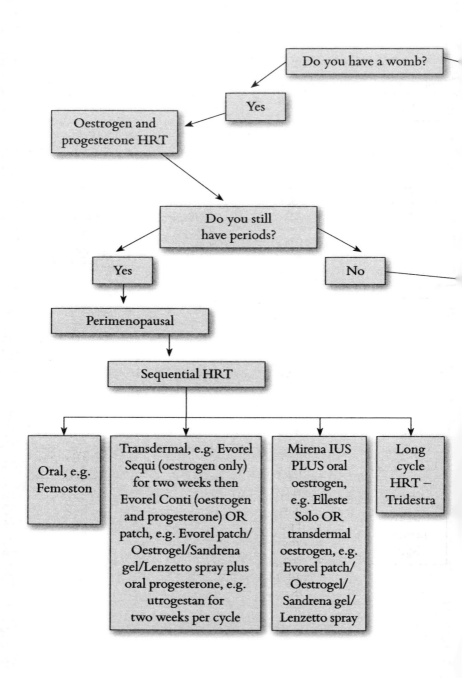

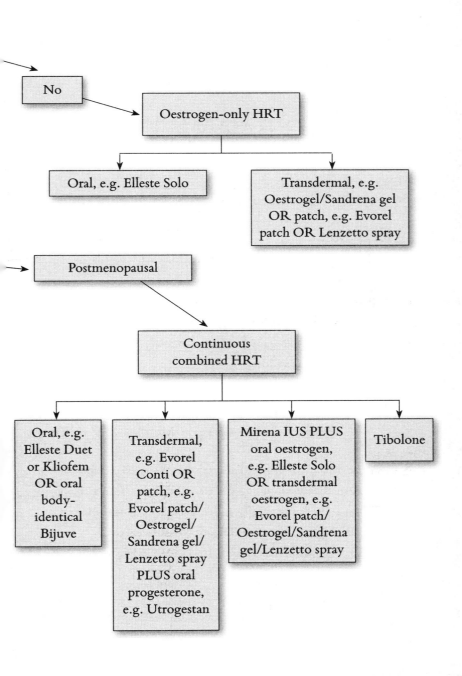

# CHAPTER 12:

# HRT – PANACEA OR BIG BAD WOLF?

———◆———

## Is HRT safe?

Here we are, at probably one of the reasons why you bought this book, at the big question – should I take hormone replacement therapy (HRT)? And I am going to put my answer out there right at the top. For most people, if you are suffering, on balance the answer is yes! HRT is not the big, bad baddie that many people thought, or still think, that it was and is.

*"I am so confused: is HRT safe? Should I be taking it?"*

Zoe, 49

So why the furore? In order to answer that we need to look back at the history of the development of HRT. HRT has been available in the UK since 1965. Originally called Premarin, it was made from the urine of pregnant horses (PREgant MARe's urine).

In 1993, the Women's Health Initiative (WHI) began a trial that looked at the effects on health of HRT, of differing types, compared to a placebo. Then, in 1996 in the UK, the Million Women Study started to collect questionnaires on HRT and its effects on health. In 2002, the Women's Health Initiative stopped part of its study due to safety concerns about breast cancer, heart disease and other health issues. The results of both studies were then published in 2003, but there was no clear guidance as to what doctors and women should do, with many women being told to stop taking HRT. In the next four years, the number of users of HRT fell from 2 million in the UK to less than a million over concerns about its safety.

In the following years, more and more research was carried out showing the health benefits of HRT. Within a few years scientists involved in the Women's Health Institute trial published further analysis of the data showing that there are additional benefits in starting HRT to those less than ten years after the menopause, including decreasing the risk of heart disease. However, they did show that there is a generalized increased risk in starting HRT after the age of 60. Now, remember that the average age for the menopause in the UK is 51, so that means starting HRT nearly ten years after the menopause.

There is lots of science out there, some good and some bad, so it is important to look behind the headlines at the structure of the study, what it was and what it did. The WHI study was flawed. Essentially it was comparing apples and oranges; the women in the WHI study were on average 63 years old, and yet in the UK most women do not have over a ten-year gap between the menopause and starting HRT. We simply cannot extrapolate the data – we cannot use the data for women over the age of 60 to assess risk for those under the age of 60. Many of the women in the study had obesity, or were smokers, both of which are risk factors for developing cancer. Two of the authors of the trial even recently published an apology in the *New England Journal of Medicine* as to how the trial was interpreted and the detrimental effect it had on prescribing rates.

Since then there have been further studies looking at the potential risks and benefits of HRT. The National Institute of Clinical Excellence (NICE) in the UK looked at all the available data and safety concerns, and guidelines were produced about the menopause and HRT in 2015, with other updates and quality standards since then and a further update due in August 2023. And yet, many women, and even some doctors, are still scared of using HRT, leading to many women continuing to suffer.

The bottom line is this:

For most women under the age of 60 who have symptoms relating to the menopause or perimenopause, the benefits of HRT generally outweigh the risks.

And to break it down further:

◆ Under the age of 50 – the benefits of HRT outweigh the risks; after all, you are simply replacing the hormones which would be expected to be present until the average age of the menopause, 51.

◆ Between 50–59 – the evidence is that the benefits of HRT generally outweigh the risks.

◆ Between 60–69 – the evidence is that the benefits of starting HRT (and the key word here is starting) are about equal to any risks.

◆ After the age of 70 – the evidence is that the risks of starting HRT in this age group generally outweigh the benefits.

# Why isn't HRT widely prescribed?

If we know the answers about safety, why aren't more women coming forward and asking for HRT? Why aren't more doctors recommending it?

The answer is complicated, and neither patients nor doctors should be blamed, and indeed the number of prescriptions for HRT has risen significantly. It is possible to become a doctor and have studied very little about HRT, though the new Women's Health Strategy aims to introduce mandatory specific teaching on women's health for medical students. Not all GPs will have done a hospital job covering gynaecology, and even if they have, this still may not have been related to the menopause. All doctors must undertake annual continuing professional development (CPD), i.e. they must continue to show that they are learning and keeping up to date with new research and guidelines. This is monitored by an annual appraisal and five-yearly revalidation process, where it is checked that all doctors have met the appraisal requirements. But changes to practice take time, and although doctors must complete CPD they can choose the areas they would like to learn about. And if patients aren't coming forward asking for HRT, perhaps some doctors are not actively searching for information about it. So, more education for healthcare professionals, doctors, nurses, pharmacists and medical students is required and hopefully will improve the situation, as will more women talking about it and asking for it, which then encourages their doctors to investigate and learn more about the subject! We all need to keep talking about the menopause and about HRT. HRT is often perceived as a complex issue, which may make some doctors feel anxious about prescribing it.

*"My friends were horrified when I said I was taking HRT. They asked me if I had read about it and told me it couldn't be safe. But I couldn't cope and was prepared to take any risks so was delighted when my doctor reassured me it was safe for me to take. Now my friends are gradually asking more and more questions as they are suffering too."*

Alex, 50

The media, both in print and on social media, also has had and continues to have a role to play. Health-scare headlines sell papers; after all a headline stating that HRT doubles, triples or even quadruples your risk of a specific disease is far more gripping and shocking than one that says, actually, it is OK. In fact, when pitching the first edition of this book, I looked and looked for similar titles, and found a wealth of books on natural solutions to the menopause, but very few on HRT! And scary stories stick – think about the long-lasting issues and concerns that people have with the MMR vaccine, despite any links to autism or other diseases being thoroughly and resoundingly disproven. This means that if you are suffering with menopausal symptoms and mention them, or HRT, to friends or family, you are, anecdotally, still more likely to be met with advice against HRT rather than for it. Which is why getting the message out about the safety of HRT – via books, media articles and documentaries – is so important. We need to change the headline so that women can get the help and treatment that they need.

Finally, I sometimes get asked whether or not doctors have misled women, whether it is as safe as we now think it is, or even whether or not we actively harmed women by giving or not giving it. Although there are exceptionally rare cases of a doctor actively trying to harm their patients, those stories make headlines for a reason – they are rare. Most of us are simply trying to do our jobs to the best of our abilities, trying to help people as much as we can and in order to do that we look to the evidence base. We look at research, and if the research tells us that something is wrong, or not safe, then we change our practice accordingly. But as more and more research is carried out with regard to HRT, what we now know is that for the majority of women HRT is safe, and therefore we must again change practice to allow women to access it.

# The benefits of HRT

*"I don't really care about anything else but stopping the flushes and being less irritable or crying less. But it is a bonus that there are other benefits too!"*

Anna, 51

### Symptom control

Let's start with the obvious – HRT works! It is effective versus all the symptoms of the perimenopause and menopause – sweats and flushes, insomnia, mood swings and irritability, joint aches and pains, tiredness, difficulties with memory and concentration, vaginal and urinary symptoms. For many women, it works. This shouldn't be underestimated!

## Protection against osteoporosis

HRT reduces the risk of developing osteoporosis, a condition where the bones become thin (more information on pages 202-210). HRT actually treats osteoporosis as well, but there are alternative treatments for osteoporosis available, so it generally isn't used primarily as a treatment. The evidence is that HRT prevents a fall in bone density and decreases the risk of fractures related to osteoporosis. Women taking standard dose HRT in the Women's Health Initiative Trial had a third fewer hip and spine fractures than those not taking it; this is a decrease from 15 fractures per 1,000 women to 10 fractures per 1,000 women on a placebo.

## Dementia

Oestrogen seems to be protective against dementia, particularly Alzheimer's dementia. There have been multiple studies regarding HRT and dementia and the results have sometimes been contradictory. The current evidence suggests that HRT is not a treatment for dementia once it has developed but that if started within ten years of the menopause it is likely to be protective against it.

In 2019, a study was reported in the media that HRT increased the risk of dementia. However, this was an observational study that simply looked at people and it could not make any statements about cause. The numbers involved were small, there was no mention of testosterone, and the study didn't report about the different ways of delivering HRT.

Other studies have shown that HRT is actually protective against dementia and testosterone is known to be protective in the brain against a form of damage called oxidative stress and other forms of damage. For example, a study showed that HRT is associated with less shortening of telomeres (the end of chromosomes) in women who carry a particular gene (APOE-e4) that is associated with developing Alzheimer's disease. In 2021, a huge study was released where the health records of over 400,000 women were studied, and this showed that HRT is associated with a lower risk of dementia as well as a reduced risk of developing multiple sclerosis. It is thought that the key is the timing of taking HRT – that taking it early, perhaps in the perimenopause, is thought to be protective, before brain changes are made.

Currently, the balanced view is actually that HRT is protective against dementia – however, HRT should not currently be started solely in order to prevent dementia.

## Other benefits

- There is evidence that HRT is also protective against osteoarthritis, the degenerative "wear and tear" arthritis associated with increasing age.
- Other possible benefits shown in studies include protection against colorectal cancer, reducing cases by approximately a third, from 16 per 1,000 women to 10 per 1,000 women on HRT.
- It may also protect against eye conditions such as cataracts and macular degeneration.
- There is some evidence that HRT may improve muscle mass and strength, which also decrease with age.
- It also improves the quality and condition of your skin and hair, and, while some doctors consider these issues to be superficial

or simply cosmetic, for some women they have a big impact on their mental well-being. HRT is not started solely for cosmetic reasons, however.

- There are also the knock-on effects of HRT which could be considered to be beneficial. For example, if you sleep better, feel less tired and your joints don't hurt you are much more likely to exercise which will help prevent cardiovascular disease.

- Cardiovascular disease – can be put in both the benefit and risk boxes. If started within ten years of the menopause, or before the age of 60, HRT does not increase the risk of heart disease. There is also evidence that it can be protective for the heart, especially oestrogen-only HRT.

- Remember, although these are potential added benefits of HRT, current guidance does not suggest that HRT should be prescribed to try and prevent these conditions.

*"Oh the added benefits are a joy. I thought I would just stop being drenched in sweat at night, but my skin is great, I feel great and quite frankly, the sex is better than great!"*

Yvette, 53

# What are the risks related to HRT?

*"I won't start HRT, I read it causes cancer."*

Fran, 54

## Breast cancer

Many women have read the headlines in the press or have heard about the risk of breast cancer with HRT, but in fact the risks are small and many women taking HRT do not have an increased risk of breast cancer. Let's break it down clearly:

Although breast cancer is often oestrogen driven, the current research shows that oestrogen-only HRT has little effect on breast cancer. As such it appears that it is the progesterone in HRT which may be related to the breast cancer risk.

Women who have gone through a premature menopause and take HRT do not have an increased risk of breast cancer (as ordinarily you would expect to have these hormones until the average age of the menopause at age 51). Here, years of HRT exposure would only be counted after the age of 50.

Taking HRT of oestrogen and micronized progesterone (Utrogestan) is not associated with an increased risk of breast cancer for the first five years and even after that point there is only limited evidence of a small increased risk.

Combination oestrogen and progesterone HRT (using non-micronized progesterone) is associated with a small increase in breast cancer (after one year of use). The key here is "small".

HRT does not affect your risk of dying from breast cancer. Importantly, if you do get breast cancer it is likely to be better differentiated. This means that the cells look more like breast cells, as opposed to poorly differentiated, which means the cancer cells are dividing quicker and therefore more mistakes are being made, so the cancer cells look less and less like breast cells. A better differentiated cancer is easier to treat, so although HRT does not affect your risk of dying from breast cancer it may well make it easier to treat.

Of the progesterones used in HRT, micronized progesterone in the form of Utrogestan has the lowest risk, and remember the risks are small! The risk associated with combined HRT is similar to that if you drink approximately two glasses of wine a day or are overweight. Remember that there are factors that decrease the risk; exercise, for example, reduces your risk of developing breast cancer!

There you have it: yes, combined HRT is associated with an increased risk of breast cancer, but that risk is small, smaller than obesity and comparable to other lifestyle factors. Looking at the information you might think that it would therefore be better to take oestrogen-only HRT, but it is known that if you have a womb, taking oestrogen-only HRT increases your risk of womb cancer.

And one more point: after you stop taking HRT, the risks are related to the length of time on HRT, and in time return back to the level of someone not taking it. This suggests that HRT does not initiate breast cancer, rather that it may promote (in a very tiny way) abnormal cells which are already present.

*"I thought it caused breast cancer in huge numbers, in fact I think I even told friends it did and not to take HRT. When my doctor explained the numbers I was really surprised and felt I had been misled by what I read, and more worryingly had then passed that onto my friends. I had to correct that!"*

Georgina, 52

## Endometrial/womb cancer

It may seem to make sense that if oestrogen-only HRT decreases your risk of breast cancer that it should always be used. But oestrogen-only HRT stimulates thickening of the lining of the womb and increases the risk of endometrial or womb cancer, doubling it from two per 1,000 women aged 50–59 to four per 1,000 women after five years' use; but increasing by much more to 32 women per 1,000 after ten years of use. Therefore, if you have your uterus you will always be offered combined HRT containing oestrogen and progesterone. There is also evidence that offering continuous progesterone in the form of a Mirena IUS decreases the risk of endometrial cancer better than sequential progesterone. Any use of an IUS decreases your risk of developing endometrial cancer by almost 20%.

## Ovarian cancer

Some studies have been inconclusive, some showed no increased risk with HRT, while the Million Women study suggested a slight increased risk. Current data suggests an extra one case per 1,000 women, but more research is needed as currently there is no good-quality evidence with respect to ovarian cancer and HRT.

## Cardiovascular disease – heart disease/attacks and/or stroke

After lots of analysis and studies it is now thought that:

◆ Your risk of cardiovascular disease is dependent on lots of other factors, including your age, weight, blood pressure, whether or not you have high cholesterol, diabetes and more, before considering any effect HRT has on it.

- Starting HRT before the age of 60 does not increase your risk of developing cardiovascular disease and recent research has shown that it may actually be protective for the heart. This is not the case for starting after the age of 60, but this is not common practice in the UK. Using transdermal oestrogen and micronized progesterone in the form of Utrogestan is the best combination to protect your heart.

- If you get cardiovascular disease, HRT has no effect on whether you die from it or not.

- HRT taken orally in tablets does slightly increase the risk of stroke. BUT, that risk is still very small in women under the age of 60, and, importantly, taking HRT in the form of patches or gels does not affect stroke risk.

- It is thought that if HRT is started early, before the lining of the arteries becomes thickened, that it could help prevent heart disease, though more research needs to be done.

## Blood clots – venous thromboembolism

Blood clots can occur in the legs (deep vein thrombosis or DVT) or in the lungs (a pulmonary embolism) or in the brain.

- Taking oral HRT tablets causes an additional two cases of blood clots per 1,000 women aged 50–59 (without HRT the number of cases is five per 1,000).

- The risk is greatest in the first year of using HRT and in women who have other factors for developing a clot, such as a family history, a clotting disorder, smoking, or obesity.

◆ However, delivering the oestrogen component of HRT transdermally, through the skin via a patch or gel, is not associated with an increased risk of clots.

### If transdermal oestrogen is safest, why have other options?

Put simply, the tablets came first and still exist and your preference is taken into consideration. Some women dislike the idea of patches, gels or creams, or don't get on with them for a variety of reasons, so the oral option is still available. And now there is a body-identical oral form of continuous combined HRT (Bijuve), which is lower risk than other oral forms (see page 236).

# Weighing up risks vs benefits – how to decide

*"I have read so much information that I feel more confused than before, should I take HRT or not?"*

Hattie, 49

*"I read a lot, then I spoke to my doctor and had a lot more questions. I read the leaflets she gave me and then went back with more questions. The more I research, the more comfortable I am with my choice."*

Agatha, 52

Everything in medicine, or indeed in life, is a balance between the potential benefits and potential risks or side effects. Even something as simple as putting on a plaster, or taking over-the-counter paracetamol could lead to an allergic reaction or even anaphylaxis. However, for most people this risk is small when compared to the potential benefit of the plaster applying pressure to stop bleeding or covering a wound to prevent infection, or the benefit of the paracetamol to relieve a headache or other pain. So, too, the risks and benefits of HRT can be weighed in the balance.

*"HRT changed my life. Actually, it is more than that, it saved my life. My relationship, my ability to work, my friendships, myself. This outweighs anything else."*

Louise, 53

Personal choice of course matters, and for each woman that may well be different, with a different emphasis on what matters most. However, from a medical point of view, looking at the evidence, it is possible to produce the following general guidelines, as described at the start of this chapter.

These are generalizations and your own medical history may affect the choices made:

- Under the age of 50 – there are no risks associated with HRT at this age, as it replaces the hormones normally expected to be present until the average age of the menopause, which is 51 in the UK.
- Women who start HRT within ten years of the menopause, and then continue to take it in the long term, have a lower risk of all causes of death, including cancer.
- Ages 50–59 – the benefits of starting HRT generally outweigh the risk.

◆ Ages 60–69 – the benefits of starting HRT are approximately equal to the risks.

◆ Over the age of 70 – the risks of starting HRT generally outweigh the benefits.

But there are choices in the route and form of HRT which reduce even these small, known risks:

◆ Starting HRT within ten years of the menopause, or before the age of 60, can help protect against cardiovascular disease (see page 211) and dementia (see page 258).

◆ Using transdermal oestrogen via a patch or a gel decreases the risk of clots.

◆ Using micronized progesterone is associated with lower breast cancer risk.

◆ A Mirena IUS for continuous delivery of progesterone gives additional protection against endometrial cancer.

*"I wish I hadn't waited as long as I did to take HRT, worrying about cancer risks. Once I spoke to my GP and understood these risks were really small, there was no stopping me!"*

Grace, 52

*"My GP was really good at explaining risks, small as they are, but for me, even if those risks were bigger I was prepared to accept them, I could not have continued as I was."*

Francesca, 54

*"I wish that there was more in the papers about how small the risks are, especially about breast cancer. I thought they were much bigger but when put in context they really aren't. Why isn't there more out there about this? Why are we suffering when the pros of HRT far outweigh the cons?"*

Imogen, 55

## Can everyone have HRT?

Not quite, there are a few contraindications, or reasons why you would not be prescribed HRT. Some of these are obvious – you can't have HRT if you are pregnant for example. Other reasons include undiagnosed abnormal vaginal bleeding such as bleeding in between your periods or after sex, a current or recent blood clot in the leg or lungs, a current/recent heart attack or womb cancer. If you are being investigated for suspected breast cancer, or if you currently have breast cancer, whether or not you are being treated for it, and if you have a liver disease causing current abnormal liver function tests your doctor may avoid prescribing HRT. Uncontrolled high blood pressure is also a reason to avoid HRT, though it can be started when the blood pressure is under control.

Having one of these issues doesn't mean that you will never be able to have HRT. For example, if you have abnormal vaginal bleeding and the cause, such as a polyp, is found and treated, you may then be able to have HRT. Or, if your liver disease is treated, or brought under control so the liver function tests return to normal, or depending on the disease itself, your doctor may ask for advice from a gynaecologist as it may be that delivering the HRT transdermally, avoiding the liver, would be appropriate. So although there are some contraindications, they may not affect you permanently!

And if they do, then we do have prescribable alternatives to HRT available (more information in Chapter 14).

Some specific conditions:

◆ Migraines – having migraines, with or without aura, is NOT a contraindication for HRT, though migraines with aura are a contraindication for the combined hormonal contraceptive pill. This means that if you have migraines with aura you will not be able to use the combined pill as a form of HRT until the age of 50, but you are still able to use both sequential and continuous combined HRT. The advice given to doctors when prescribing HRT for patients with migraines is to use body-identical transdermal oestrogen, so deliver with a patch or a gel, use the lowest dose of oestrogen to control symptoms and if progesterone is needed use a Mirena IUS, micronized progesterone as in Utrogestan, be it via pills or pessaries, or other oral progesterone or through the skin in combined patches.

◆ Breast cancer – if you have or have had breast cancer or are at high risk of it you may be offered alternatives to HRT (for more information on prescribable alternatives to HRT please see Chapter 14). If you have one first-degree relative (mother, sister) with breast cancer over the age of 40, or two second-degree relatives (aunts) at any age you are considered to have the population background risk of breast cancer. Taking HRT doesn't lead to any extra risk of breast cancer because of your family history, only the very small additional risk from the HRT itself. So if your mum had breast cancer at age 42, 50 or 60, it is not a contraindication to you having HRT. If you are at higher risk of breast cancer, or carry the BRCA1/2 gene then you may wish to consider alternatives to HRT.

◆ Obesity – you should be offered transdermal oestrogen in order not to increase the blood-clot risk.

◆ HIV – the advances of HIV treatment with antiretroviral therapy has meant that people with HIV who are stable and on treatment have an average life expectancy, so more women are going through the menopause with HIV. There is no contraindication to having HRT with HIV.

◆ Other health conditions – depending on your past medical history and any other medication you take, certain preparations of HRT may be more appropriate than others. For example, if you have a history of liver problems, or gallstones or are taking medications that affect liver enzymes (e.g. some anti-seizure medications) you may be advised that the transdermal route is the most appropriate.

*"I was upset when I went to the doctor for HRT and she asked me about bleeding in between my periods and then wouldn't give it to me because I did have bleeding in between! But she found chlamydia on my swab, and I am so glad she treated that. Now I am on HRT, and STD-free!"*

Bridie, 49

*"I didn't ask for HRT as I knew I couldn't have the contraceptive pill because I have migraines with aura. I was so surprised and grateful to be wrong!"*

Peace, 52

## SUMMARY POINTS

◆ HRT has various benefits in addition to improving symptoms, such as promoting bone health.

◆ The risks of HRT are small and can often be decreased by changing how the HRT is delivered. For example, the risk of blood clots is reduced by delivering oestrogen through the skin as opposed to orally.

◆ In women under 60, the benefits of HRT in general outweigh the risks. Between 60 and 70, the benefits and risks are approximately equal, and after 70 the risks may begin to outweigh the benefits.

# CHAPTER 13:

# HRT – THE PRACTICALITIES

---◆---

## How to start HRT

After taking your history your doctor will take your blood pressure. If this is high it will need to be brought under control before starting HRT in order to decrease your risk of cardiovascular disease. Once you are ready to start HRT, if you are starting a sequential form of HRT you will start the oestrogen component within five days of starting your period. Then you roll the packs together continuing on to the next as you finish your first. If you are having an IUS inserted and you are still having periods, it is best to fit the coil during your period (as your cervix is slightly open making it easier to insert, and because we know you aren't pregnant at that point!), but it can be inserted at any point as long as there is no risk of pregnancy. If you no longer have periods, continuous combined HRT can be started at any point. If you are using sequential HRT you can manipulate the timing of the withdrawal bleed by delaying taking the two weeks of progesterone. However, this is not recommended either regularly or for more than one to two weeks as otherwise essentially you would be taking oestrogen-only HRT which is associated with an increased risk of endometrial cancer.

For more information about how to use patches/gels please see page 247

## Does it work straight away?

That depends. For some women, their sweats or flushes reduce quickly, within a few days, but it often takes three to four weeks, though the maximum effect can take up to three months or so. Other symptoms such as insomnia tend to improve within three months of starting. You may also find that any initial side effects (see page 275) settle down within three months. In general, a preparation will be used for three months before changing.

*"I thought it would be like taking a painkiller, that my symptoms would just vanish. It took a while and weirdly it was only when I was asked a few weeks later that I realized that I hadn't had a flush. I always noticed flushing but hadn't really noticed the absence of hot flushes, I just went back to normal."*

Promise, 53

## It isn't helping – now what?

It can take a few months to see the full effects of HRT so your doctor is likely to encourage you to wait three months to see if your symptoms improve. If there is no improvement, generally the oestrogen component can be increased from the starting dose. For example, the dose of Oestrogel tends to start at two pumps of gel per day but women may need anything from one to four pumps to achieve symptom control, or, more rarely, and off-licence, at higher doses. (Off-licence use here means that the manufacturer of the medication has not applied for a licence to either use the medication for this condition or at this dose.)

*"I waited for things to get better, I was hoping they would, but it wasn't the cure-all I thought it would be. So I stopped taking it. It was only when I went to the GP for something else and he asked me about it that I said I stopped because it didn't work. He changed the formulation, wham bam, goodbye aches and pains, hello good sleep!"*

Janey, 49

Before increasing the dosage your doctor will check that there aren't reasons preventing you from receiving the full dose. For example, if you have a bowel condition meaning that you aren't absorbing the full dose orally, you may have better control using a transdermal route; or if you find that the patches aren't sticking (which is rare) you may want to try an alternative patch or another delivery route. It is also important that your doctor checks that there isn't another reason why your symptoms aren't improving, such as a thyroid problem. Some people will absorb better with one preparation than another.

Finally, and this is important to say (but potentially difficult to hear, or in this case read), HRT helps symptoms that are related to low levels of oestrogen, but if you have a symptom not related to this, or your tiredness or irritability are due to another cause, it won't help!

*"I thought HRT was the cure all, and that life would suddenly get better. My friends would say it was life-changing. It wasn't, it wasn't that it didn't*

*work, it did and sleeping better, being able to concentrate at work and not having sweats helped me deal with life better, but it didn't solve the depression I have suffered with for years. It was only then that I went to the doctor for help with my mood."*

Sandra, 50

# Side effects

*"Oh, it was like having PMS all over again, my boobs were so tender!"*
Eva, 51

As discussed above, everything in medicine is a balance between benefits and potential risks and side effects, and medicine can have side effects! With regard to HRT, many women find that the side effects settle down, so doctors normally encourage you to wait for three months to see if they do disappear on their own. But if they don't then please do speak to your doctor as there are options available. Firstly, the doctor needs to work out which hormone could be the culprit for your side effects. If you are taking oestrogen-only HRT this is pretty easy, it can only be the oestrogen! But if you are taking combination HRT it can be either hormone – or both – causing the issue, or it can be related to the way of delivering the medication.

## Bleeding
◆ Some 85% of women taking sequential HRT will have a monthly withdrawal bleed. This is not a side effect but a result of hormone withdrawal.

◆ Some women on sequential HRT will have irregular or heavy bleeding but this tends to settle down within approximately three months. If it doesn't, tell your GP; it may require investigating or an alternative such as a Mirena may be advised.

◆ Continuous combined HRT often leads to irregular bleeding or spotting for the first six months. If it persists, or starts after six months, again tell your GP who will investigate possible causes.

## Side effects from oestrogen

◆ Breast tenderness, fluid retention, leg cramps or pain, bloating, headaches, feeling nauseous, indigestion.

◆ Options to treat these include reducing the dose of oestrogen (as long as symptoms are still controlled), changing the type of oestrogen being used and changing the route of delivery of the oestrogen.

◆ Breast tenderness can also be treated by rubbing a non-steroidal inflammatory gel (such as an ibuprofen gel) into the breasts.

◆ Nausea can be helped by taking oral HRT at bedtime instead of in the morning, though again changing to a transdermal route can also work.

## Side effects from progesterone

Progesterone intolerance, or progesterone sensitivity, is when you are extremely sensitive to the hormone progesterone. There are two main types of progesterone: body-identical, or micronized progesterone, which is made from yams and has the same chemical structure as the progesterone made naturally by the body. The second type is progestogen, which is a synthetic form of progesterone that, although similar, is not structurally the same as that made by your ovaries. Progestogens are found in contraception and in some forms of HRT. Progestogens are more likely to lead to progestogen intolerance than progesterone, which is also safer.

Symptoms of progesterone intolerance include acne, breast tenderness, bloating, headaches, fluid retention and fatigue, as well as anxiety, mood swings and irritability and low mood. These symptoms can also occur initially with progesterone but may often settle down.

If you have a womb you will need to take progesterone as part of your HRT to keep the lining of the womb thin and decrease the risk of womb cancer. Depending on whether you still have periods, you may be given progesterone either cyclically for two weeks each month, or at a lower dose daily. Some people find that they have fewer symptoms related to progesterone intolerance when they are on the lower daily dose of a continuous combined regime than when they were on a sequential form.

**What can be done?**

If you are on a synthetic progestogen then changing to body-identical micronized progesterone (Uterogestan) may help with symptoms. If not, then it may be possible to change how you take the progesterone, for example swapping from using it orally to vaginally, though this is an off-licence use of the medication. Alternatively, you could use the Mirena IUS, which may still cause side effects similar to pre-menstrual syndrome, although these often settle down within a few months.

## Side effects from a patch itself

◆ Some patients report irritation from the patch. This can be treated by ensuring that you change the application site of the patch frequently, or by using a different route, e.g. a gel instead of a patch. Another option is to use a steroid inhaler, just like those used in asthma, to calm down the inflammation under the patch. Using a steroid cream may mean that the patch doesn't stick but puffing the steroid inhaler onto the skin before applying the patch is often really effective!

◆ Other patch issues – the patches tend to stick well, even when showering or swimming, but sometimes they may leave a sticky mark when they are removed, although adhesive remover wipes and sprays are available. Some women report that if you put them under the edge of clothing or a belt that the edges may roll a little bit but they don't come off. If you find that they aren't sticking well (which is unusual), wiping with an alcohol wipe and ensuring that there is no cream/lotion on the skin before applying may help.

And one my patients worry about, no matter the medication, and which in this case is a myth – weight gain! While the menopause often results in weight gain, HRT does not!

*"It took some time but we got the balance right in the end, but even if we hadn't, I was prepared for tender breasts before my bleed, it would have been worth it to avoid all my other symptoms, but changing the progesterone helped."*

Sonya, 50

# Why might I be referred to a menopause clinic?

There are various reasons why your GP may refer you to a specialist menopause clinic, which could either be run by a GP with a special interest (and qualifications) in the menopause or by gynaecologists. Before that point, though, there may be a particular GP in your practice that you can see who has experience, and sometimes additional qualifications, in the management of the menopause.

You may be referred before starting HRT if you have a history of a hormone-dependent cancer, such as hormone receptor positive breast cancer, or if you have a complicated medical history. Once you have started HRT you may be referred on for various reasons: if your symptoms are not well controlled, despite increasing dosage or changing route of delivery; if you have persistent side effects despite manipulating the hormones and route of delivery; if you have an increase in how heavy or the length of your bleeding on sequential HRT, or the bleeding becomes irregular, or if any bleeding on continuous combined HRT lasts for over six months, or starts again after six months. So if it isn't working, or you aren't tolerating it, then your GP will refer you to a specialist.

However, there are not many specialist menopause services in the country, so you may have to wait, or may be referred to a general gynaecologist in the first instance if required.

*"I was lucky, my GP didn't say no to HRT, she prescribed it. But no matter what she did I still didn't feel right, either there were side effects or it didn't seem to work. I saw a gynaecologist who added in testosterone, and suddenly I felt like me again."*

Magda, 56

## Monitoring on HRT

As with many medications you will need to be monitored while on HRT. Generally, the first review is three months after starting the medication, or three months after any change in the HRT. The purpose of this consultation is to assess how effective the HRT is, to ask about bleeding and any other side effects and to check your blood pressure. If adjustments are made then you will be offered a follow-up appointment after a further three months.

Once you are settled onto the correct regime for you and are happy with your symptom control you should be reviewed once per year. At this appointment, again the doctor or nurse will check the HRT is still working effectively for you, without intolerable side effects. Your blood pressure will also be checked. Every year the healthcare professional will also discuss with you the benefits and risks of HRT, so that you can decide each year, weighing up any other changes in your medical history or other factors, to see whether or not to continue with it, or if changes are required. For example, after the age of 60, it is recommended to use a transdermal form of oestrogen rather than a tablet form as the transdermal form is not associated with any increased risk of blood clots.

*"I was used to going to the GP surgery every year for my pill check, so now it was once a year for my HRT check – simple!"*

Esme, 53

# Can HRT stop working?

If you start HRT during the perimenopause or early in the menopause then you are likely to still be producing some oestrogen, so you may only need a low or starting dose of HRT to control your symptoms. Over time it can seem that the HRT stops working, that your symptoms return, but actually it is not that the HRT isn't working, rather that you are producing less natural oestrogen and therefore need higher doses of HRT in order to replace it and get the symptoms back under control. Increasing the dose of oestrogen in your HRT doesn't affect the risk of breast cancer, but if the oestrogen is taken orally it may increase the risk of deep vein thrombosis (blood clot). As such, delivering the oestrogen transdermally is a safer option. There is a minimum amount of progesterone required for womb protection. An increase in oestrogen dose may not always be required: sometimes changing the preparation, e.g. gel to cream or vice versa, can somehow increase the absorption of oestrogen and improve symptoms.

# How long can you take HRT for?

*"Each year I get anxious that they are going to say I am going to have to stop taking it."*

Madhvi, 62

There isn't an arbitrary stopping point or limit to how long you can take HRT for; you don't have to stop after one, two or ten years! In fact, people can continue to take HRT for as long as they feel it is beneficial or useful for them to do so. Indeed, this is part of the purpose of the annual HRT check, to check that the need for it and its benefits still outweigh the risks. While the recommendations are for women to take it for the shortest time required, each woman will have symptoms for differing lengths of time so will need HRT for differing lengths of time, meaning some women will continue taking oestrogen in their 60s, 70s and beyond. The benefits of symptom control and to prevent osteoporosis will continue but the balance of the risks may become greater depending on your history.

For vaginal oestrogen, there is no long-term risk, it can be used for long-term maintenance indefinitely, as long as you don't have active breast cancer.

*"I will continue for as long as I feel I need to, or am able to, I feel well and recognize myself on HRT. When I wasn't on it, I felt unwell and exhausted all the time."*

Zoe, 58

## Stopping HRT

If you do decide to stop HRT, or it is recommended that you do so, your doctor will generally advise that you gradually decrease the dosage to try to stop symptoms returning. If you stop suddenly the oestrogen levels will fall rapidly, which can trigger symptoms again. Depending on the dosage of oestrogen you are taking this slow reduction can take a few months. So your doctor may switch from a high-dose oestrogen to a standard dose for two or three months, then to a low dose for another few months, before using oestrogen on alternate days for a period of time before stopping. Decreasing this slowly can help reduce any flushes or other symptoms but that may still occur. You may find that your symptoms return after stopping the HRT but they may subside and settle, so you may be advised to wait a few months before deciding whether to remain off HRT or start it again. If you are struggling with vasomotor symptoms of flushes or sweats you may be offered alternatives to HRT.

Remember, though, that if you no longer have symptoms such as flushes or insomnia and don't need HRT for these, if you do develop genitourinary syndrome of the menopause (see page 169–175 for more information), you can start vaginal oestrogen at any point and continue it forever, without risks.

*"I will admit that I was really anxious about stopping, and when I had my first flush after stopping I was petrified I was about to be thrown back to the horror of my late 40s, but actually I only had a few and they went away pretty quickly."*

Precious, 60

# Bio-identical vs body-identical HRT

*"I didn't want to risk any of the risks of HRT. I thought that by having bio-identical HRT I was doing the safer thing."*

Tara, 53

This is a controversial area of menopause management and HRT. There are various clinics offering what is called bio-identical HRT, often stating that these are natural, more effective and safer than traditional HRT, with fewer side effects. Sounds good so far, right? These bio-identical, or compounded hormones (also called compounded bio-identical HRT, or cBHRT), are made from yams and have the same chemical structure to the hormones found in the body. The clinics make up the combination of different hormones which they believe will be effective, individually for each patient, compounding the medications together.

But so does body-identical HRT (also called regulated bio-identical HRT rBHRT), which has the same chemical structure to the hormones found naturally in the body and is also made synthetically from plant chemicals found in yams or soya beans. And we can alter the dosage of hormones as needed, using an oestradiol as the form of oestrogen and micronized progesterone which are identical to the hormones in the body.

The issue here is one of safety: the individual components of bio-identical HRT may well be safe but the bio-identical preparations are not regulated in the same way as medications are (by the Medicines and Healthcare Products Regulatory Authority MHRA) as they are considered to be natural supplements, so they may contain uncontrolled or unregulated amounts of hormones. Some bio-identical HRT clinics use measurement of hormone levels in your saliva to decide how much hormone to give, but these levels fluctuate depending on the time the test is taken and your diet and don't correlate with the levels of hormones in other parts of the body nor the amounts required to relieve symptoms.

There is little research to suggest that salivary hormone levels are useful, therefore they generally aren't taken in the NHS. There is also limited evidence of efficacy, for example with regard to bone protection, or safety data about these compounded hormones.

HRT is also often made from natural products (in fact many medications are), but it is regulated and controlled. In 2017, the Advertising Standards Agency ruled against a clinic regarding misleading promotions of bio-identical compounded hormones, leading to a ruling that clinics should not claim that compounded bio-identical HRT is more effective or safer than regulated HRT as there was no evidence to suggest this, nor was there evidence that using salivary hormone tests were an effective tool to personalize any treatment. Does it work? Quite possibly, though the data used is that extrapolated from regular HRT, but that also means that it is subject to the same risks and side effects as regular HRT. In some circumstances, women are prescribed progesterone creams which don't seem to be absorbed well by the body.

Put simply, there isn't the data to show that bio-identical HRT is effective, or safe, and it is currently unregulated. (For more information on complementary and alternative options, see Chapter 15.)

*"I was at a dinner party and the topic came up. One of the women who I didn't know was a GP and when she said that you can get body-identical HRT on the NHS I was so surprised, and then grateful when she explained more. I thought I was being safer, but perhaps not. I saw my own GP and now have a prescription for regular HRT."*

Ellie, 53

# HRT shortages

In recent years, since the first edition of *The M Word* was published, we have had multiple HRT shortages, of various items from patches to gels and more. This came to a head in the first half of 2022 when there was a severe shortage of Oestrogel and other products, which then led to a domino effect meaning that many people could not get their HRT (see the introduction, page 15). The impact of people not having their HRT cannot and should not be underestimated. For many people, it enables them to stay healthy, in themselves and in their relationships, and to remain in work. The HRT shortage caused significant anxiety for many people, as well as taking up a lot of time in GP surgeries and pharmacies.

There were stories of people paying extortionate prices at online private pharmacies, buying HRT on the black market rather than using reputable pharmacies, sharing with friends, using out-of-date medications, and even travelling to buy HRT abroad. This is clearly far from ideal, or even safe; friends may not be on exactly the same treatment as you. Even if the bottles and boxes look similar, what is right for them may well not be the right treatment for you. Getting medications abroad means that the patient information may not be in English or in a language you understand, so you may not be receiving what you think you are. This also means that your doctor won't know what you are taking, so there can't be effective or safe monitoring, or follow-up.

While the government and pharmaceutical suppliers work to resolve the HRT shortage crisis, it may be useful to have some information in case a shortage arises again in the future. The main point is that you do not need to stop your HRT or ration it out in order to make it last longer as there are likely to be prescribable alternatives to the HRT you are already taking. Rules have also been put in place so that pharmacists can substitute prescriptions with a suitable alternative.

So your GP may be able to prescribe, or your pharmacist supply, an approximately equivalent HRT until any shortage is resolved. You may find that you get different levels of absorption between different methods of delivery of HRT, with some women responding well to a low-dose preparation in one form but needing a higher dose preparation of another, so you may choose to go back to your original prescription once any shortage is over. The information below may also be useful when moving abroad, or even to different parts of the UK that may have alternative prescription guidelines, though there is a drive from menopause campaigners for a national prescribing list so that everyone has access to the same medications.

The following are approximate equivalent dosages of transdermal (delivered through the skin) body-identical oestrogen, called oestradiol.

It is also worth noting that some women find that higher doses of the Lenzetto spray do not absorb as well into the body.

|  | Gel – Oestrogel | Gel – Sandrena sachets | Lenzetto spray | Oestrogen patch |
|---|---|---|---|---|
| Low dose | 1 pump | 0.5 mg | 1–2 sprays | 25 mcg |
| Medium dose | 2 pumps | 1 mg | 2–3 sprays | 50 mcg |
| High dose | 3–4 pumps | 1.5–2 mg | >3 sprays | 75–100 mcg |

- If, for some reason, no transdermal equivalent is available, then your GP could consider an alternative HRT such as Bijuve, which is a form of body-identical combined HRT and as such has lower risks than other forms of oral HRT. Alternatively, oral HRT is also an option, with 1 mg oral oestrogen being considered an equivalent for low-dose HRT, 2 mg oral oestrogen for medium-dose, and 3 mg oral oestrogen for high-dose HRT.

- There are also alternative versions of progesterone available if needed. Uterogestan is a body-identical micronized progesterone, while other preparations are slightly different but will also give womb (endometrial) protection – essential if you are taking HRT and have your womb.

- Uterogestan 100 mg orally = 5 mg Provera orally = 5 mg Norethisterone orally.

- Alternatively, a Mirena intrauterine system (coil) can also be used for womb protection. It also works for contraception and for treating heavy menstrual bleeding, which can occur during the perimenopause.

- With regard to vaginal oestrogen, there are various options including Ovestin cream, Blissel gel or Imvaggis pessary, which all contain the oestrogen estriol; and estradiol pessaries, tablets (Vagifem), and the Estring, which all contain estradiol.

- Whatever the situation or shortage, there may be equivalents available, so please speak to your GP.

## SUMMARY POINTS

- There is no time limit for how long you can have HRT.

- Dosages may need adjustment over time, either increased, decreased or stopped.

- Compounded bio-identical HRT is not regulated by the MHRA, while regulated body-identical HRT is available and has efficacy and safety data.

# CHAPTER 14:

# SO MANY CHOICES...
# PRESCRIBABLE
# ALTERNATIVES TO HRT

———◆———

*"I wanted HRT, I hoped for HRT, but I couldn't have it as I had breast cancer last year. But thankfully instead of me slinking out the room in the depths of despair, and dripping with sweat from the current hot flush, my GP said we still had other choices, thank God for that!"*

Aliyah, 51

There are various reasons why you may not be prescribed HRT, such as the medical contraindications listed on pages 268-270, personal choice, or having tried it but not liked or tolerated it, perhaps due to side effects. But there are still lots of other choices available to treat your symptoms, with evidence to say that they are effective. Lifestyle measures are covered in Chapter 4 and complementary therapies are covered in Chapter 15, while this chapter focuses on prescribable alternatives to HRT. HRT can improve all symptoms of the menopause, from the vasomotor symptoms to fatigue, joint pains, brain fog and more, as well as being beneficial for bone health. The prescribable alternatives to HRT have generally only been tested for their impact on the vasomotor symptoms of hot flushes and sweats. Some of these alternatives can also help with mood symptoms including irritability, anxiety or low mood.

Which one to try or use depends on your symptoms, medical history and other medications you may be taking, so it isn't quite as simple as start with X and if it doesn't work try Y, as your treatment will be individualized to your needs. The current guidance on treatment of the menopause doesn't recommend using these medications for the menopause but your doctor may consider them. The first line of treatment for menopausal symptoms is HRT, but there are other treatments available.

*"I just don't want it. The doctor tried to convince me about the safety of HRT but I just don't want it, or at least I want to try an alternative first. But I still want something that works."*

Lilly, 52

# Clonidine

Clonidine is a medication which is used to treat high blood pressure and to prevent recurrent migraines as well as treating hot flushes. It works by affecting the thermoregulatory centre in the brain, making it less sensitive to tiny changes in temperature and hopefully therefore treating flushes. It is licensed for use in the perimenopause and menopause to treat hot flushes; the other meds in this chapter are not licensed for this use but are used this way. However, although it is licensed for hot flushes, current guidance states that it should not be used routinely to control symptoms.

Clonidine is generally prescribed for a two- to four-week trial, the dosage varies between 25 mcg and 150 mcg per day (generally either as 50 mcg three times a day, or 75 mcg twice a day).

## Side effects

Side effects are common; about one in two women on clonidine will describe some sleep disturbances such as insomnia, nightmares or unusual dreams. Other side effects can include tiredness, nausea, dry mouth and constipation. As the side effects of clonidine are common, it isn't often used for hot flushes, though it can be. Higher doses tend to be more effective, but they also may have more side effects. If it hasn't worked after a four-week trial then it should be stopped and an alternative considered.

## Contraindications

If you have a low baseline blood pressure it may not be suitable as it can bring down your blood pressure further. If you have high blood pressure it can help with this or work in conjunction with other high blood pressure medications, though it can interact with some of these medications. Other contraindications to clonidine include a low pulse rate due to specific heart rhythm abnormalities. It should also be used with caution if you have a history of depression.

*"It sounded like a good option for me and it definitely helped bring down my blood pressure which had been too high. But unfortunately I exchanged hot flushes for a constant dry mouth and feeling sick. Out of the frying pan and into a very dry-mouthed fire. Next!"*

Natalie, 49

# SSRIs – antidepressants

*"I have lots of symptoms I admit, but depression isn't one of them. Why am I being given an antidepressant?"*

Tanya, 52

SSRI stands for selective serotonin reuptake inhibitor, which is a class of drugs licensed for use in depression and anxiety. These work by increasing the levels of serotonin in the brain. They also have an effect on the thermoregulatory centre in the brain and so can be effective in treating hot flushes. They seem to work for 20–50% of women who have flushes, whether or not you have depression and anxiety. They also can have a positive effect on mood, anxiety and general well-being. Depression and anxiety are common symptoms of the perimenopause and menopause but the first line of treatment for these symptoms is still HRT, unless these conditions predated the perimenopause/menopause.

SSRIs include paroxetine, citalopram, escitalopram, fluoxetine and sertraline. The evidence is that the best option for the treatment of hot flushes and sweats is paroxetine, working for about 50–60% of women.

*"I know that my mood isn't good and that I am so much more irritable than I used to be, but I really think that I am not depressed, I never have been before and the only thing that has changed is that I can't sleep. I was surprised when my GP asked about my periods, I had no idea that this could be because of the menopause, or that HRT might help."*

Michelle, 51

## Side effects

Side effects of all SSRIs include nausea, dry mouth and dizziness, which tend to settle down after the first couple of weeks. They can also cause a worsening of symptoms initially, including anxiety, and although sertraline is particularly good to treat anxiety it is also most likely to cause an initial worsening of symptoms, which tend to last a few days. Other side effects which may not tail off include sleep disturbances and sexual dysfunction such as difficulties reaching orgasm and decreased sex drive. But while SSRIs can take a few weeks to reach full effect with regard to improving mood, they tend to work much quicker – in just a few days – for hot flushes and sweats, so your doctor may give a trial of one to two weeks. If you wish or need to stop an SSRI you will need to reduce it gradually over a period of time, to prevent any withdrawal symptoms such as headaches, sweating, worsening of anxiety and nausea, but if you only used them for a trial period of one to two weeks this weaning down period is generally not needed.

*"I didn't want to use HRT and my doctor suggested paroxetine for my hot flushes, even though I wasn't depressed. It did work for me and interestingly I also feel much more evened out in general."*

Michelle, 50

## Contraindications

If you have had breast cancer and are taking tamoxifen, then you should not take the SSRIs fluoxetine or paroxetine as these can interfere with its efficacy. However, other SSRIs can be used.

*"Breast cancer is a b\*tch, first you have breast cancer, which is bad enough, then I had surgery and radiotherapy, which weren't that much fun. I already had hot flushes from the menopause but when I was put on tamoxifen they got worse. But I can't have HRT and then my doctor said I couldn't have the antidepressant that my friend was on for her flushes. So yes, breast cancer is a b\*tch. My doctor didn't give up though, she did some research and found that I could have sertraline, which helped a bit, they made the hot flushes much less frequent."*

Emily, 54

# SNRIs – antidepressants

SNRIs are selective serotonin and noradrenaline reuptake inhibitors, which do as they sound, they increase the levels of serotonin and noradrenaline in the brain. Venlafaxine is generally used to treat vasomotor symptoms, and works for 20–60% of women. Again, they also have an antidepressant effect and can improve mood and quality of life.

## Side effects

The side effects of venlafaxine can be more pronounced than with an SSRI, though the side effects are similar including dizziness, headache, insomnia, sweating and sexual issues. However, there is no interaction with tamoxifen so can be used if you are taking it after breast cancer.

## Contraindications

SNRIs should not be given with poorly controlled epilepsy or if you have been diagnosed with bipolar disorder and are in a manic phase.

*"Even if I hadn't had breast cancer I know that I wouldn't have been keen on HRT, no matter how safe it is. I just didn't like the idea of adding hormones when my body wasn't producing them. But I also wasn't keen on the flushes. My GP and I tried a few things but venlafaxine worked for me, I took it for about 18 months and then gradually came off it. And now I don't have any symptoms at all."*

Pam, 56

# Gabapentin

Gabepentin is a gamma amino-butyric acid analogue (try saying that ten times in a row!) which is used as an anti-seizure medication to treat epilepsy as well as being used to treat nerve (or neuropathic) pain, such as pain during or after an episode of shingles, and to prevent migraines. Studies have shown that when used at doses of 900 mg per day they can reduce hot flushes for about 50% of women. It also works to help insomnia and improve sleep, which can also be problematic in the menopause, and can help with aches and pains.

## Side effects

Side effects include increased appetite, weight gain, drowsiness, fatigue, rashes, ankle swelling, dry mouth, tremor and dizziness. But the risk of these side effects can be reduced if it is started at a small dose and then increased gradually to reach an effective dose. All the side effects with gabapentin tend to improve with time. If you do decide to, or are advised to stop taking gabapentin, you will be advised as to how to slowly reduce and wean the dose down over time to prevent any withdrawal effects. Don't stop taking it suddenly.

## Contraindications

Although not contraindications, gabapentin should be used with caution in patients with a history of mixed seizure epilepsy, psychotic illness or substance abuse.

*"I had a bout of shingles which caused a hugely painful rash in a band over the left side of my back and tummy. But when the rash went away the pain did not and after trying various meds my doctor started me on gabapentin. And within a few days all my hot flushes vanished, killing two birds with one stone!"*

Priya, 53

# Pregabalin

Like gabapentin, pregabalin is used to treat epilepsy and neuropathic (nerve) pain, as well as being licensed for use in anxiety. It is about as effective as gabapentin, working to treat hot flushes in about 50% of patients and can also lead to improvements in mood and well-being.

## Side effects

Pregabalin can cause the same side effects as gabapentin including weight gain and drowsiness, though these seem to be less severe than with gabapentin, so pregabalin tends to be well tolerated. Just like with gabapentin, pregabalin should not be stopped suddenly and needs to be weaned down slowly.

## Contraindications

There are no absolute contraindications, but pregabalin should be used with caution in patients with a history of substance abuse or severe congestive heart failure.

*"To be honest, I thought it was HRT or nothing, so I didn't even ask for anything. Turns out I was wrong!"*

Dalia, 51

# Cognitive behavioural therapy

*"I already thought I was losing my mind, and then the doctor said he wanted to refer me to see a psychologist. So I must be going crazy, right?"*

Farrah, 50

Nope, not right! Your doctor discussing cognitive behavioural therapy with you is not a sign that they think that you are crazy, though actually doctors tend not to describe their patients as crazy in general! The NICE guidance regarding the menopause recommends that GPs and other healthcare professionals discuss cognitive behavioural therapy with their patients, to help with menopausal symptoms.

## What is cognitive behavioural therapy?

Cognitive behavioural therapy (CBT) is a form of psychological, or talking therapy, which is effective in treating lots of conditions, from anxiety to low mood, panic attacks and chronic pain. The cognitive part is the thinking bit, the thoughts that we have, while the behavioural part is the behaviours that come from it. For example: I have anxious thoughts, so I avoid whatever is making me anxious; the thought led to the behaviour. But then the behaviour feeds back into the thought, so if I avoided what was making me anxious, I must have done so because it is something to be worried about, so I become more worried about it!

We all have multiple thoughts and stories in our heads, some of which are useful and helpful, others of which are not. CBT aims to help you understand and work out which of your thoughts are helpful and that you should engage with, and which ones are not so useful, so you can learn not to engage with them. It is a skill, which takes time and practice. If you put all your unhealthy thoughts in a box in your head but need to spend all your time sitting on the box to stop those thoughts coming out, you really are still engaging with them. The skill is to accept that those thoughts are there and let them pass you by. Which is easier said than done, especially when your thoughts are still racing at two in the morning and you just can't turn your head off!

Acceptance and commitment therapy is a form of psychological therapy that can be useful for menopausal symptoms. This form of talking therapy focuses on accepting the emotions related to the symptoms (rather than the symptoms themselves). Accepting, as opposed to fighting, the emotions can allow people to commit to changing their behaviours if needed as well as improving their quality of life.

*"Everything is all mixed up, the more I worry about sweating, the more I sweat, the more I worry about not sleeping the less I sleep, the more I worry about failing at work, or not being a good mother or wife, the more depressed I get and then I feel I am an even worse mother."*

Frannie, 51

Let's think about this in terms of menopausal symptoms, which are often interlinked. Let's say that you are suffering with hot flushes and sweats and because of this you are worried about giving a presentation at work, or even embarrassed to socialize with your friends. This may lead to you starting to avoid those things, just in case a flush happens, but this can then worsen stress and low mood as well as feelings of anxiety. Add into the mix the sleep problems which are so common around the menopause, and the stress, anxiety and depression can get worse, as can difficulties with memory and concentration. Put in simpler terms, the worry and stress over any symptom, from brain fog to sleep, can worsen the symptom, which in turn worsens the stress and anxiety! The same can apply to low mood and depression; the negative thoughts that you have about yourself lead to low self-esteem, which may prevent you performing as normal, at work, or in relationships, which then makes your mood even lower. So there is a two-way street between the mind and the body and the body and the mind and all the symptoms involved. CBT aims to break this cycle to help you manage your symptoms.

## How can CBT help?

With regard to the menopause, CBT is offered, and can be effective for: anxiety, stress, low mood and depression, insomnia and other sleep problems and even for vasomotor symptoms. CBT specifically aimed at menopausal symptoms can help you manage them better, even those you traditionally might think are more physical such as hot flushes and sweats, and the improvements seen in these symptoms in trials of women having CBT were maintained even six months after the course of CBT was finished. CBT is effective, but it isn't a magic pill, it takes time and practice to work, but it really does work!

*"To be honest, I went because my husband said I had to go. I didn't think it would work, I didn't think anything would work really. And I was embarrassed to talk about it in case the person judged me. But they didn't and little by little, over time I was able to see things differently."*

Zara, 52

## How do you get CBT?

CBT can be delivered in a variety of different ways, via books, apps, online courses and face-to-face sessions delivered by healthcare professionals including doctors, counsellors and psychologists, be they group sessions or on a one-to-one basis. Your GP may be able to refer you, or depending on your area you may be able to self-refer, often online, to local NHS psychological therapy. Some courses such as Moodgym or Moodjuice are available online, CBT-based apps such as Sleepio are also available, though a fee may be charged.

*"I was really surprised when my son said he used an app to help him sleep, but to be honest I was willing to try anything by that point, including being bashed over the head with a club each night, just to get some sleep! But it really worked, and I am less grumpy because I am less tired, and can exercise again, because I am less tired and am not sure I should admit it, but I think I am a nicer person because I am less tired!"*

Mai, 47

# What is next?

Research is ongoing and there are some developments with regard to a group of medications called PhytoSERMs. SERM stands for "selective oestrogen beta receptor modulator", and the phyto means from plants. This complicated name essentially means that the medication aims to be selective, in that it may stimulate or simulate the effect of oestrogen on the brain and the rest of the body but NOT on the breasts and reproductive organs. We very eagerly watch and wait for further news and developments.

Finally, let's not forget the impact of non-prescribable options such as exercise, which are beneficial in so many ways! For more information please see page 116.

## SUMMARY POINTS

◆ If HRT is not suitable other treatments are available depending on your symptoms.

◆ HRT is the first line treatment for menopausal symptoms.

◆ Hot flushes can be treated with various medications including a medicine used to treat high blood pressure, anti-epileptic medications and antidepressants – note that these aren't to treat epilepsy or depression, but to treat the vasomotor symptoms.

- Cognitive behavioural therapy can be an effective treatment, not just for psychological symptoms but also physical ones such as hot flushes.

# CHAPTER 15:

# WHAT ELSE IS OUT THERE?

———◆———

Some of my patients feel that the menopause is a natural part of a woman's life and that this means that they should either not treat it, or deal with it "naturally". However, as with everything in medicine, we must weigh up the risks, benefits and reasons for coming to a choice. We could even start with whether or not the menopause is indeed natural, or is a by-product of us living far longer than we have previously ever done, so perhaps it isn't natural to live for 30 years or so after your periods have stopped. Getting pregnant and giving birth is natural, and even disease processes such as a heart attack are not unnatural, but medical professionals would encourage you to have monitoring and treatment if needed for these as well. However, I totally understand that many patients would like to try a natural approach, either in the first instance, or alongside other measures. Indeed, taking a holistic approach to medicine, or in this case the perimenopause and menopause, is the most effective for patients, so lifestyle measures (covered in Chapter 4) should always be advised and discussed as part of a treatment plan.

As a doctor, trained in Western medicine in the UK, I am not at all "anti" complementary treatments or medicine. I practice what is known as "evidence-based medicine", which is medicine where we have evidence of efficacy and safety. This isn't always possible with herbal or complementary therapies, which either may not be suitable for a randomized controlled trial, or there may not be the funding available for such trials to create the evidence that many medics are looking for. But this doesn't mean that they won't work for you, and like many doctors, I support my patients in using complementary therapies, not alternative ones. This is because "complementary" implies the two forms, both traditional Western medicine and the complementary medicine working together (or at the very least informing each other of what is being offered), while "alternative" suggests closing down one avenue altogether. If it works for you and is safe, then that is brilliant, we are all after the same aim — for you to be symptom-free, well and healthy.

## Are "natural" remedies safe?

In order to show evidence that a medication or remedy works, it needs to be statistically significantly more effective than a placebo, which essentially is a dummy medication that contains no active ingredient. The "placebo effect" is real, with patients in studies into various health conditions, not just menopausal symptoms, reporting improvement in their symptoms when taking a placebo — the belief that the medication will work, makes it work. Alternatively, it is possible that symptoms improve naturally with time, and this may also be relevant with regard to menopausal symptoms. But it may not even be possible to do a trial against placebo for some alternative remedies; for example, you would know if you had acupuncture or a massage-based treatment or not! For each of the options discussed below, the evidence for them working is covered.

A word of warning, though: natural does not necessarily, or always, mean safe. We have obtained our medicines from plants for thousands of years; for example, aspirin comes from willow bark, digoxin from the foxglove plant and certain forms of HRT from yams! So although we may now make something synthetically it can still be derived from a plant. This means that we know that plants and herbs are effective. But it also means that they can have risks and side effects when interacting with other medication. So if you are taking any herbal medication please do inform your doctor.

A second issue is around the regulation of herbal remedies, which have not previously had the same level of regulations as other medications, meaning that you could not ensure that each pill or tea contained the same amount of the relevant herb. There is now a regulatory system in place in the UK, the Traditional Herbal Medicine Scheme (THR). If you see the THR symbol on herbal medicine you therefore know that it has been subject to stringent regulations, that each tablet contains what it says on the label, at the dosage stated on the label. The label should also list any potential side effects or interactions with other medications. As such it is safer to only use products which have been approved and regulated by the Traditional Herbal Medicine Scheme, with the THR logo/ symbol on the label.

*"I thought that natural meant safer, but I developed terrible itching after starting a remedy, so I must have been allergic to it, just like I could be to any medicine."*

Sandra, 53

*"I have always tried to treat things with my diet and herbs, I don't like using painkillers to hide pain but want to treat the reason for it, same with the menopause, I will use herbal remedies if I need to."*

Agata, 49

# Phytoestrogens

Phytoestrogens are naturally occurring oestrogen-like compounds which are found in plants. As such it is thought that they can act like oestrogen in the body, and therefore may help with menopausal symptoms. Women in countries where the diet is naturally high in phytoestrogens – found in foods such as soy beans, eaten commonly in Japan – seem to have fewer symptoms during the menopause, particularly vasomotor symptoms, and have lower rates of heart disease, and breast, womb and colon cancer. So it would appear that eating a diet rich in phytoestrogens could help stave off symptoms as well as having a long-term beneficial health effect, though there may well be other factors involved in reducing symptoms. There is some evidence to show that phytoestrogens reduce hot flushes, though other evidence suggests little effect. What also isn't known is whether this kind of diet needs to be eaten over your whole life, or at least a prolonged amount of time, or if any long-term benefits can be obtained from eating them for a shorter period of time, or starting later, such as when symptoms start.

PhytoSERMs are supplements that are being researched currently and contain particular phytoestrogens. For more information please see page 302.

*"I don't know if it was the phytoestrogens in my diet which helped or the fact that by trying to eat more of them I was eating healthier food in general and a lot more fruits and veg. I lost weight and felt better. Win, win really!"*

Shalini, 54

## Where can I find phytoestrogens?

Supplements are available, or you can adapt your diet to increase the amount of phytoestrogens you eat. These are found in soya beans, soy products such as tempeh (though not soy sauce!), some seeds and legumes such as linseeds, lentils and wheat berries, fruit and vegetables such as yams (from which we derive much of HRT), strawberries, beansprouts, tomatoes. For more information about phytoestrogens, how much to eat and more, please see page 307.

Red clover is a herb which contains isoflavones, which are phytoestrogens. As such red clover is often marketed for treating hot flushes and menopausal symptoms. The evidence is mixed, with some studies showing benefits but many showing no effect. Women who have or have had breast cancer, are taking tamoxifen or have other hormone-dependent cancers such as womb cancer should avoid phytoestrogen supplements including red clover as it is possible that they could have an effect on the cancer returning. More research is required.

# Herbal remedies

Herbal remedies are those made from plants and are available in health food shops and pharmacies. Remember that we obtain many of our medications from plant sources so the fact that something is herbal, or natural, does not mean that it is safe! If they work it is because there is something in them. There are various herbal remedies that have been considered useful for menopausal symptoms which are discussed below.

## *Agnus castus*

Also known as chasteberry, agnus castus can be used as a tablet or a tincture (where the herb is dissolved in alcohol). It is used for multiple women's health issues such as period pain, heavy periods and pre-menstrual syndrome. Although often promoted for use in the perimenopause and menopause, there is little data available regarding its effectiveness on specific menopausal symptoms.

## Black cohosh

Also known as *Cimicifuga racemosa*, bugbane, or black snake root, though it is a plant not a snake; the root of it is gnarled and black, so perhaps looks like a curled up black snake. It was traditionally used by Native Americans to help with labour and period pains. It seems to affect serotonin levels in the body, and we know that medications affecting serotonin can help with hot flushes but also mood changes; however, there is no evidence that it is effective for menopausal symptoms. There previously were concerns about liver toxicity with black cohosh but that is now thought to be related to contaminants in the products; high-quality extracts of black cohosh have not been shown to affect the liver, but it is recommended to avoid them if you have active liver disease, or known liver damage.

*"This was the one I had heard of, so I tried it, for about three months, didn't make things worse, but didn't do much either. But my friend swears it stopped her flushes."*

Elsie, 53

## Sage

The herb sage, which you can grow in a pot on a window sill, is traditionally used to treat hot flushes. Commercial teas containing sage extract are available, though some people simply steep the leaves in hot water. Sage extract is also available as a tablet. Research is ongoing into the effectiveness of sage, but there is some evidence to suggest that sage supplements may help with hot flushes and sweats. Again, if you are taking tamoxifen your doctor may advise you to avoid sage, which can also be an issue with high blood pressure, as it may increase the blood pressure or interfere with high blood pressure medications.

## Wild yam

This would seem to make the most common sense; if scientists manufacture HRT from yams why not just take yam extract supplements, or use a cream containing wild yams? But there isn't evidence that this works; the body cannot break down the yam into the oestrogen and progesterone needed.

*"I like yams, so I ate them, and I used yam cream on my body. And then I also went to the doctor!"*

LaToya, 52

## Other herbal remedies

Other herbs are available which have been marketed for use in women's health, though not always specifically for the relief of menopausal symptoms, or for specific symptoms which may, but not always, be due to the menopause:

- Evening primrose oil – often promoted for breast pain and mood changes or mood swings related to PMS, but there isn't sufficient evidence to suggest that it can help with these or with other menopause symptoms. Can lead to skin rashes and nausea.

- St John's wort – also called *Hypericum perforatum*. Is effective for anxiety and depression, but interacts with many other medications such as the oral contraceptive pill and antidepressants. Please check with your pharmacist or doctor before starting. Also remember that the current guidance suggests that if anxiety or depression start during the perimenopause or menopause that antidepressants should not be given first line, but to consider HRT instead. So if this is extrapolated, St John's wort should also not be given primarily to treat anxiety and depression which starts related to the menopause.

- *Ginkgo biloba* – reputed to improve circulation and aid memory. Not proven to be effective in memory or concentration difficulties related to the menopause. Must not be taken with drugs that prevent blood clotting such as warfarin as it can increase their effects and increase the risk of bleeding.

*"It was only when I started taking St John's wort and started feeling a bit better that I realized how bad I had been. I told my doctor and she referred me for some talking therapy as well. Not sure which helped more, but it has worked."*

Rose, 48

## Bio-identical hormones

Bio-identical hormones are often promoted as a natural alternative to HRT. For more information please see page 283.

## Other complementary therapies

There are many forms of complementary therapies, involving massage, exercise and much more. Some complementary therapies which have been promoted as useful for menopausal symptoms are covered here. While it may be difficult to obtain evidence of efficacy for these treatments they may well have added value in that they can be relaxing and reduce stress. Indeed, the opportunity to talk to a professional for an hour about your symptoms and concerns can be helpful in itself. It may be that why it works, or how it works is not as important as whether or not it works for you.

## Why does it matter if there is evidence that it works?

How much it matters whether or not it works depends on the reasons you are looking at a treatment. If as a patient you have found a form of therapy, of whatever kind, and you find it effective and can afford to have the treatment then the evidence in general probably matters less. But if you are the National Institute of Clinical

Excellence setting guidance for doctors about which treatments to try first, the evidence base definitely is important, as is the safety data. And then decisions are made about the cost effectiveness of treatments, especially if they are being considered to be available on the NHS. While every patient matters there are a finite amount of funds available and deciding on the cost effectiveness is a significant medical ethical issue.

The bottom line is this, if it works for you, and it is safe, then you must do what helps you! Just please do always tell your doctor. Complementary medicine should be just that: complementary, running alongside Western medicine – or at the very least let us know!

● Traditional Chinese medicine – can involve a combination of herbal medicine, acupuncture, massage and exercise such as tai chi. Acupuncture is also used by medical doctors, for example to relieve pain, and involves inserting very fine needles into the body in specific places depending on the symptoms experienced. There is some evidence to suggest that acupuncture may help with hot flushes, but the study did not compare it to a placebo group (because this would not be possible with acupuncture; you know if you have had the needles inserted or not!).

● Ayurveda – a traditional system of medicine from India, involving herbal remedies, diet changes, massage, meditation, yoga and exercise. There are some studies which show the benefits of yoga for menopausal symptoms such as insomnia, but again it is not possible to have a placebo-controlled trial, as you would be aware if you were practising yoga. You may find that massage and meditation are helpful to relieve stress and promote relaxation, which can be very helpful.

- Magnet therapy – magnets are thought to promote healing and balance the nervous system. Some women report that wearing a magnet on their underwear, such as the LadyCare device, reduces menopausal symptoms, though there is no evidence to support this finding.

- Homeopathy – involves diluting a plant or herb, often one which has similar properties to the symptoms you may be having, to minute amounts. Many of the herbal products described above will be available as homeopathic remedies. There is no official evidence to support their use, but they are unlikely to cause harm.

- Reflexology – involves massage to the feet, applying pressure on specific points thought to be related to or correspond to different body parts or bodily functions. Again, there is no traditional evidence that this is effective, but it is very difficult to obtain a randomized controlled trial, you will know if you have had a session of reflexology or not! Patients often describe reflexology as relaxing which has its own benefits!

- Aromatherapy – this involves using essential oils from plants, either in the bath or with massage. The practitioner chooses the oil or mix of oils depending on your symptoms, for example lavender is thought to help with insomnia and sleep and chamomile and geranium to help with anxiety or to help you feel calm. There is little evidence of efficacy, but also little evidence of harm!

*"I just feel better, more like myself, or who I used to be. And whether it is the massage, the essential oils or the opportunity to relax, spend time on myself or the chats about anything I like with the therapist which is helping, I can't answer. I just know I feel like me again."*

Cara, 49

## SUMMARY POINTS

- There are many complementary therapies available, and many claim that they improve menopausal symptoms.
- It can be difficult to carry out randomized controlled trials to prove efficacy for many complementary treatments.
- If you are going to use a herbal remedy, look for the Traditional Herbal Registry (THR) mark to ensure that the product is regulated.
- Always inform your doctor of any herbal remedies or complementary therapies you are taking/having as there can be interactions with other medications.

# THE MENOPAUSE TOP TEN: ANSWERS TO COMMON QUESTIONS

———◆———

These are the ten most asked questions about the menopause – hopefully, a quick "dip in" resource for you!

## 1. What is the menopause?

The menopause means the last period, and is a diagnosis of hindsight! You are not postmenopausal until you have not had a period for 12 months. Any bleeding after that point is considered to be postmenopausal bleeding and needs assessment by a doctor.

## 2. How can I have symptoms when I still have periods?

The menopause means the last period, and the perimenopause is the period of time leading up to that point, which can last a few years. You can have symptoms during the perimenopause, whether or not your periods are regular or irregular. Importantly, you can still get treatment, irrespective of whether or not you still have periods!

### 3. What are the symptoms of the perimenopause/menopause?

There are lots of symptoms of the perimenopause and menopause and these can be divided into physical symptoms and psychological or mind/mood/mental health symptoms. Physical symptoms include changes to your periods, hot flushes and sweats, joint pains, palpitations, headache, insomnia and loss of libido. Symptoms related to mental health include low mood, anxiety, depression, irritability and mood swings, and brain fog. For more information about symptoms please see Chapter 4.

### 4. Will I definitely get symptoms and when?

Approximately four out of five women will get some symptoms, and about one in four are severely affected by symptoms. As to when, the average age of the last period is 51 in the UK, and the perimenopause starts in the few years before that, commonly after the age of 45. The symptoms of the perimenopause can occur anything from a few months to ten years before the menopause and symptoms tend to last an average of four years after the last period, though can last approximately a decade. But symptoms can start earlier or later. Premature menopause (primary ovarian insufficiency) can occur before the age of 40 and some people may not have symptoms at all.

### 5. How do I know if my symptoms are bad enough to need a doctor?

There is no definite answer to this question as it is extremely personal and will change for each individual. I generally advise that if your symptoms are serious enough to be bothering you, or are having an impact on your life in some way, then that is the time you should bother me as your doctor!

### 6. If I am in the perimenopause, do I still need to use contraception?

Yes, there is still a chance of pregnancy in the perimenopause and, depending on the age at which you have your last period, after the menopause as well. If you have your last period under the age of 50, you should continue to use contraception for two further years. If you have your last period over the age of 50, you are advised to continue using contraception for one year. Irrespective of whether you are still having periods, all contraception can be stopped after the age of 55 as the risk of pregnancy is considered so small. This advice only applies to contraception for pregnancy as sexually transmitted infections can occur at any age!

### 7. What has happened to my sex drive and why does sex hurt?

Libido, or sex drive, is an extremely complex process which has both physical and psychological components. It is common for women to experience a loss of libido around the perimenopause and menopause and there are multiple reasons for this, from changing hormone levels affecting libido, to mental health symptoms affecting libido, or to physical ones, such as sex becoming painful. Genitourinary syndrome of the menopause can lead to vaginal and vulval dryness/soreness and irritation that can make sex painful. There are lots of treatment options for genitourinary syndrome of the menopause so please see your doctor. For more information please see Chapter 5.

## 8. Is HRT safe?

The general consensus is that for most women who start HRT within a decade of their menopause, the benefits of HRT outweigh the small risks. The benefits of HRT include symptom control, which cannot be underestimated, as well as decreasing the risk of conditions such as osteoporosis and colorectal cancer. HRT isn't prescribed solely for preventative reasons however. There is a small increased risk of breast cancer, but this is similar to the risk related to drinking two glasses of wine a day, and is lowest with micronized progesterone – in fact, with oestrogen-only HRT, the risk may be decreased. Other risks associated with HRT, such as blood clots, can be mitigated by changing how the HRT is delivered because transdermal oestrogen (through the skin) is not associated with increased clot risk.

## 9. Can I have HRT given my (family) history?

If you had particular types of migraines you may not have been able to use the combined oral contraceptive pill, but migraines are not a contraindication for HRT. HRT is also not contraindicated if you have diabetes. If you have had a blood clot in the past, you can still have transdermal HRT. With regard to a family history of breast cancer, having one first-degree relative (mother or sister) who had breast cancer over the age of 40, or two second-degree relatives (aunts) who had breast cancer at any age, you are considered to have the background population risk for breast cancer and can have HRT. Your doctor will ask questions to assess your individual risk and then discuss if HRT is appropriate and the safest way of delivering the medication – which is generally through the skin. Lots of women who think they can't have HRT, perhaps if they have obesity or a history of clots, can still have treatment.

### 10. What other options are there if I don't want/can't have HRT?

If you choose not to use HRT for any reason, there are other treatment options available. These include using antidepressant or anti-seizure medications; prescribing these doesn't mean that your doctor thinks you have depression or epilepsy as these medications can be used for perimenopause and menopause symptoms. Other options include cognitive behavioural therapy or making lifestyle modifications, which can be really effective, for example reducing caffeine, alcohol and stress while increasing physical activity.

# AFTERWORD

◆

There we have it, a run through of the perimenopause, menopause and health beyond the menopause and the available treatments. But perhaps the most important aspect is one not yet mentioned, and that is our mindset. Our mindset to become empowered about this part of our lives, to rule rather than be ruled by our symptoms, and to share our knowledge with others.

Menopause is not a pause, a stop or an ending. It is a beginning. A beginning of a new phase in your life where you can be in control of your health and your body and continue to be who you want to be, or do something else entirely. It is an opportunity, to take stock of your physical and psychological health, to take control of your diet and lifestyle and to move on in a new, positive and healthy way.

Since *The M Word* was published, I have done countless press interviews, podcasts and more, and I often end with a piece of information that, quite honestly, I regret not putting in the first edition of the book; in fact I generally say that as well! And it is this...

While I was researching *The M Word* and exploring why the menopause occurs, I came across an example of menopause in the animal world that to me represents how thinking about the menopause has changed in recent years. As time went by I could no longer remember which insect this story referred to, wondering if it was a cricket, locust or grasshopper. Actually, this is the story of a particular type of aphid. Insects don't have periods so they don't have a menopause in the way that you might think of it, but these particular aphids have a post-reproductive phase in life, just like we do. These aphids live in a gall, which is a swelling on a plant, and when the colony is attacked, let's say by a ladybird, these post-reproductive, postmenopause females defend the colony by essentially sticking themselves to the predator ladybird, thereby saving the day, though they do die alongside the ladybird as a result.

Now, if you'll excuse the anthropomorphism, consider how scientists and commentators might have described this phenomenon 50 years ago. Use your best David Attenborough voice (you know you want to!): "Here, the menopausal female aphids, past their reproductive prime, their youth and their best, have only one job left to do. In order to protect the colony, and as they no longer have another purpose, they must sacrifice their lives for the younger aphids." You could interpret this phenomenon as being an example in the animal world that the menopausal female is no longer of value.

Or you could interpret it (yes, still with lots of anthropomorphism) in this modern era, an era in which women have value at every stage of their lives, and whose worth is not linked to youth or reproductive functions, like this… "That this colony of aphids, when it is under attack, sends out its wisest, strongest, and most courageous – the menopausal female, who may have reproduced, or may not, who has learned from her younger years and is best able to defend the colony." Yes, these aphids still die, but this is my preferred interpretation and one that I can then transcribe to us – that the perimenopause and menopause allow us to enter these years, when we are the wisest and strongest that we have been, and continue to have space to grow and develop. Essentially, you get better with age!

We need to work together, as women, to support each other: pre-menopausal and post, periods or not, childbearing or not, high oestrogen levels or not, single or in a relationship, heterosexual or LGBTQ+. Whatever our age, we are all women, so let's look after ourselves, look after each other, hear us roar!

# ACKNOWLEDGEMENTS

I would like to thank my agent Jane Graham Maw of Graham Maw Christie, for her ongoing belief in me and support for over a decade! Thanks also to my editors at Summersdale, Claire Plimmer, Debbie Chapman and Lucy York, for their dedication to the manuscript. To Rasha Barrage, Victoria Garrard, Susanne Hillen, Imogen Palmer and Kate Cooper for their input into the second edition. To all the menopause campaigners working tirelessly to ensure that there is equal access to menopause support and to end the stigma of the menopause, and to all the doctors and patients who have ever taught me and continue to teach me on a daily basis, I thank you.

# INDEX

"Honest and heart-wrenching."
Holly Willoughby

# DOCTORS GET CANCER TOO

A DOCTOR'S
DIARY OF LIFE
AND RECOVERY
FROM CANCER

"The story of a woman on both sides, a doctor with a cancer diagnosis. A mum, a friend, a daughter and a GP."
Sara Cox

DR PHILIPPA KAYE

# DOCTORS GET CANCER TOO

*A Doctor's Diary of Life and Recovery From Cancer*
Dr Philippa Kaye

ISBN: 978-1-78783-813-0
Paperback

## "It's cancer."

**Dr Philippa Kaye** was 39 years old when she heard those dreaded words. The diagnosis of bowel cancer would change her life and mean crossing the divide from being a doctor to being a patient. She soon discovered that her years of training and experience had not prepared her for the realities of actually living with cancer.

*Doctors Get Cancer Too* tells Dr Kaye's moving story of being on both sides of the desk, and shares the insights she gained not only through the diagnosis and treatment but in surviving and thriving through cancer and beyond. Filled with practical advice, this book aims to make patients and their loved ones feel better understood, more prepared and less alone, and to provide solace for anyone navigating their way through hard times.

# *So*

# *Hot*

# *Right*

# *Now*

## The Little Book of
## Perimenopause

Peer-reviewed by Dr Samantha Sanders, health psychologist

**ALEX GREENGATE**

# SO HOT RIGHT NOW

*The Little Book of Perimenopause*
Alex Greengate

ISBN: 978-1-80007-709-6
Paperback

The years leading up to the menopause can be a daunting time, and one which is widely misunderstood. Fear not! This book is here to break the stigma and share the knowledge, answering the questions you've been too afraid to ask and demystifying the perimenopause once and for all.

Filled to the brim with essential information, this book will take you through all the stages and symptoms of the perimenopause right up to the menopause, so you can face this new stage of life with confidence.

Have you enjoyed this book?
If so, why not write a review on your favourite website?

If you're interested in finding out more about our books, find us
on Facebook at **Summersdale Publishers**, on Twitter at
**@Summersdale** and on Instagram at **@summersdalebooks**
and get in touch. We'd love to hear from you!

Thanks very much for buying this Summersdale book.

**www.summersdale.com**